The Human Genome
PLAYBOOK
For Disrupting Cancer

James W. Forsythe, M.D.,H.M.D.

The Human Genome Playbook for Disrupting Cancer

Century Wellness Publishing

Forsythe, James W M.D., H.M.D.
1. Health 2. Homeopathy 3. Cancer
Book Design: Patty Atcheson Melton

ISBN:978-0-9897636-4-6

Contents

Dedication Page
7
Chapter 1: My Clinic's Superior Survival Rate
9
Chapter 2: Century Wellness Clinic Leads the Way
23
Chapter 3: Dangerous Process Revealed
39
Chapter 4: Milestone Medical Advancements
45
Chapter 5: Significant Cancer Projects Generate Success
55
Chapter 6: Significant Health Care Industry Advancements
63
Chapter 7: Social Nightmares
69
Chapter 8: Mastering Human Traits
73
Chapter 9: More Potential Dangers and
Benefits: New Drugs Will Emerge
77
Chapter 10: Government Controls Your Health
81
Chapter 11: Chimpanzee Genome Project
85
Chapter 12: Various Side Projects Emerged
89
Chapter 13: The Mind-Boggling Decade of the 2020s
97
Chapter 14: Virtual Physiological Human
103

Chapter 15: Human Microbiome Project
109
Chapter 16: The Human Proteome Project
113
Chapter 17: Significant Systems Emerged
117
Chapter 18: 1,000 Genomes Project
121
Chapter 19: Researchers Target Diseases
125
Chapter 20: Personal Genomics Testing
127
Chapter 21: Creating New Drugs
133
Chapter 22: Historical Considerations
139
Chapter 23: Rapid-Fire Advancements Occur Daily
143
Chapter 24: Who Owns the Human Genome?
151
Chapter 25: Look to Century Wellness Clinic for Guidance
153
About the Author
157
Contact Information
159

Dedication

This book is dedicated to: the continued talents of Wayne and Patty Melton for providing extensive fact-finding, editing, graphic design and layout ~ noteworthy contributions that deserve my sincere gratitude; to my Century Wellness staff, without whose support and caring none of my many books would have been possible; and most of all to my loving wife, Earlene, along with our five children, and ten grandchildren ~ who all serve as my constant motivating force.

Results

show that conventional
Chemotherapy treatments
administered by
mainstream onologists
would never help one
half to two thirds of
Stage IV
Cancer patients.

1
My Clinic's Vastly Superior Survival Rate

The five-year survival rate of advanced Stage IV cancer patients treated at my clinic is nearly 33 times better than the national average in my current five-year study.

On a nationwide basis only a dismal 2.1 percent of all such patients survive after being treated by mainstream oncologists who deliver high-dose standard chemo.

By comparison, results at my Century Wellness clinic reflect a 5-year survival rate of more than 67 percent among such patients that I had treated at the time of this book's publication.

To put this into clear perspective, think of the situation this way: only two out of 100 advanced-stage cancer patients survive when treated by conventional cancer doctors. In sharp contrast, at least 67 out of every 100 similar people survive when I treat them. There are several reasons:

Unique tests: My clinic offers chemosensitivity tests that determine which types of chemo will most effectively treat a specific individual, while also identifying which drugs, hormones and natural supplements work best for the patient.

Effective process: Before treatment begins, I meet with each patient to develop an effective treatment process based largely on results of the chemosensitivity tests.

Natural treatments: My clinic uses effective and safe natural treatments that not only refrain from damaging the body, while killing cancer and fortifying their natural immunity. These are unlike dangerous drugs used by mainstream oncologists who often administer harmful synthetic substances that often damage patient health and may lead to death.

Cancer obliterated: In most cases my unique treatments generate a 90-plus-percent kill rate of the cancers within such patients. This often enables the patients' immune systems to assume and to successfully carry out the job of completing our fight against the disease, leading to remission. The natural ability of my patients to kill off all remaining cancer increases significantly when I administer superior, effective immune-boosting natural substances.

The 67-percent cancer survival rate generated by Century Wellness Clinic reflects patients who remain alive five years after treatment. Numerous survivors at that point have at least some cancer; among many of these individuals the disease is considered "manageable." Most doctors generally refer to such patients as "cured," particularly individuals who remain in remission after five years.

Consider Me Unique

My treatments sharply boost the possibility of a cure, thanks to the fact that the chemosensitivity tests specify which drugs would work best, and which would be ineffective for each specific patient.

As noted in my newsletters for patients, thanks to the chemosensitivity tests made possible by genomics research, "no other oncologist in the United States can offer this kind of information to his or her patients. What conventional oncologists offer only is what has been the best results of the latest clinical study."

Those reports, which have nothing to do with chemosensitivity tests fail to generate 100-percent accuracy. In fact, many studies embraced by mainstream oncologists are only 30 percent to 50 percent accurate in predicting outcome.

Results show that conventional chemotherapy treatments administered by mainstream oncologists would never help one half to two thirds of Stage IV cancer patients.

Sadly, these patients are merely being poisoned when given chemotherapy, which does little to eliminate cancer--while intensifying their suffering.

Consider Me A Maverick Doctor

Before initially visiting my clinic, many patients soon realize that I'm one of just a handful of working "integrative medical oncologists" worldwide.

This means that I'm fully licensed to practice medicine as a mainstream medical oncologist, while simultaneously working as a board-certified Homeopathic physician using natural treatments.

"I essentially use what some people call 'the best of both medical worlds," I sometimes tell patients. "If I'm giving you the wrong drug, I'm killing you. But that's what traditional oncologists are doing every day."

My unique Century Wellness Clinic, located in Reno, Nevada, in the western United States, fights cancer with harmless and effective natural substances. We do this without the excessive use of the poisonous, dangerous and expensive drugs such as high-dose chemo administered by mainstream oncologists.

Instead, depending on each patient's specific needs and results of the person's chemosensitivity tests, I develop individualized treatment regimens. These often include extremely limited regimens of low-dose chemo along with various natural remedies.

Sadly, mainstream oncologists are forced by the standard medical industry's required protocol to administer deadly regimens of high-dose chemo to all advanced Stage IV cancer patients--with no exceptions.

From the view of many mainstream doctors, I'm threatening to "overturn the proverbial apple cart."

Under such a scenario, would the resulting "public outcry" generate an ideal situation where frustrated patients worldwide and vote-hungry politicians insist that every mainstream oncologist order chemosensitivity tests for all cancer patients?

Patients Yearn for Effective Natural Remedies

Every week, many patients from around the world travel to Century Wellness Clinic for treatment of cancer or other ailments.

Every week out-of-state license plates are seen in my clinic's parking lot, after patients drive from as far away as Maine, Florida, Alaska, Canada and Mexico.

This influx of visitors provides a consistent and significant boost to the Reno-area economy, generating thousands of hotel room occupancy, with average patient stays at three to four weeks.

A noticeable portion of these patients from every continent except Antarctica. courageously visit my clinic, after being told by mainstream oncologists elsewhere tell to get their affairs in order.

"Never take the word of any doctor who would tell you something like that," I say to patients. "Every patient needs to remain hopeful for as long as possible."

Genetics Research Makes this Possible

Much of Century Wellness Clinic's success in effectively treating cancer patients has been made possible by genomics research, along with my previously mentioned natural remedies.

These technological advances stem from studies inspired by the Human Genome Project, when scientists mapped out the entire human genome from 1990 to 2003.

Findings made possible by genomic research since then have enabled scientists to develop the amazing chemosensitivity tests. I consider this as an essential, vital and necessary tool for cancer doctors when developing effective individual treatment regimens. Yet keep in mind that as previously mentioned, mainstream oncologists insist on ignoring these techniques.

So, as you might imagine, I've been called a "maverick doctor," largely due to my unwillingness to follow the proverbial dictates of allopathic physicians.

You see, I refrain from "following the proverbial pack" of mainstream doctors. Instead, I choose to essentially stand in my own field while proudly enabling my patients to benefit from effective new genomic technologies that other doctors ignore.

Patients Benefit From Choices

My Stage IV cancer patients at Century Wellness Clinic are given a choice regarding their own treatment regimens.

This serves as a sharp contrast from the process offered by mainstream oncologists; those physicians refuse to enable patients to make such decisions.

At my clinic, patients who wish to go conventional at least know about the best drugs for them. At that point, they then have the right answer.

We also send all patients home with the appropriate supplements deemed highly effective for their individual cancers, renewing these products on an as-needed monthly basis.

Chemosensitivity Testing Works Wonders

Every year, tens of thousands of cancer patients in the United States fail to receive genomics-generated cancer chemosensitivity tests that could save their lives.

In countless instances such procedures could prevent certain patients from receiving poisonous chemo that never would help them. When that happens high-dose chemo ravages their bodies. This invariably leads to extremely painful, horrendous and lingering death. Their bodies literally waste away.

"On a widespread social scale, this is a tragedy seemingly beyond belief," I tell patients who inquire about the issue. "The sad fact is that most mainstream oncologists either refuse to or fail to inform their patients that chemosensitivity tests exist."

From the standpoint of the vast majority of allopathic cancer doctors, everything essentially comes down to "guesswork" because of the dismal fact that they refrain from seeking such procedures.

Compounding the problem, as mentioned earlier, medical industry standards require mainstream oncologists to follow "protocol." These puzzling rules mandate that all patients with certain types of advanced-stage cancers always be given specific types of chemo drugs at a pre-designated, high-level; these are administered on pre-set schedules.

Disturbing Results Emerged

By my estimates, in the United States every day nationwide more than 1,300 cancer patients needlessly die such deaths--the equivalent of several jumbo jets crashing into the ocean.

The amount of human suffering is immeasurable on a grand scale.

Yet why do mainstream doctors refuse to recommend such tests? Does mainstream medicine's close ties with Big Pharma--the giant multi-billion-dollar pharmaceutical industry--have anything to do with such the disturbing behavior of these physicians on a grand scale?

While no one can accurately give an irrefutable answer to these critical questions, at least something is clear--patients need to be proactive.

Demand Such Tests

Any person suffering from cancer, particularly advanced Stage IV levels of the disease, should demand the option of taking such tests before any chemo begins. Here are the steps such patients should take:

Access: Before treatment begins, tell the doctor that you want a "cancer chemosensitivity test."

Options: Inquire about what options are available from the doctor for receiving such tests.

History: Ask if the doctor has ever given patients access to such procedures.

Red Flags: Be on the lookout for a "red-flag warning" that if the physician refuses to offer these tests.

Avoid Conventional Oncologists

When I tell my clinic's cancer patients about this, they immediately start avoiding mainstream oncologists--often telling many people that they know to do the same.

I have been issuing such warnings for many years.

In fact, as I noted in my clinic's October 2010 newsletter, "gene testing has the answers" for cancer patients seeking to benefit from cutting-edge technology.

From my view now in my fifth decade of practicing cancer medicine, the development of such tests emerged as "the biggest C-change in all my years of practice with more than 200,000 patient visits."

Patients Appreciate Access

At Century Wellness Clinic, the advent of cancer chemosensitivity testing has made a major difference in the lives of our patients' success levels and improved overall survival rates. These statistics became evident in our present, ongoing five-year, 800-patient study.

Drawing whole blood at my clinic, cancer chemosensitivity tests are relatively simple, easy and productive procedures. Upon their initial visits to Century Wellness, some people with cancer are what homeopaths call "virginal treatment patients."

The designation signifies that those individuals have not yet been treated for their cancers, and therefore have never been subjected to potentially dangerous or deadly treatments such as multiple drugs, radiation, or even major surgery.

For the most part upon their initial visits to Century Wellness, these patients know that their disease is advancing, and their prognosis is guarded. They know their time factors are limited and they want real answers, along with effective non-toxic treatment.

Avoid the Guessing Game

Most of them highly educated and extremely inquisitive, these patients want to avoid getting ensnared in the type of "guessing game" used by mainstream oncologists.

With equal importance, as I clearly stated in my 2010

newsletter, these patients "don't want an oncologist that picks out drugs and throws them against a wall to see if any stick in terms of their own cancer response rates."

A highly trained and experienced member of my professional staff begins the chemosensitivity testing process by taking a patient's whole blood--a very simple and easy procedure. The blood is then handled very carefully, while undergoing stringent packaging and shipping requirements; samples remain good for 96 hours prior the time when the Greek laboratory analyzes the sample.

My personnel always draw the blood on the first part of the week, ensuring that the sample gets to its destination in a safe, preserved and fresh manner.

Upon arrival at the testing laboratory, scientists and lab technicians subject the blood to high-tech tests. At last count, my clinic estimated that at least three labs provide this service--one in Germany, one in Greece and one in South Korea.

We Fine-Tuned Efforts

Following several years of testing, at Century Wellness we found that the Greek Test offers the most important information in terms of the number of chemotherapy agents and supplements that are tested along with the greatest accuracy.

To its credit, the Greek company, RGCC, Research Genetic Cancer Centre, tests at least 12 families of chemotherapy agents and 60 types of supplements.

Once RGCC receives the blood, the testing process takes from 10 days to two weeks for completion of the analysis. To do this, the lab's technicians and scientists sample and harvest the cancer cells--which are then cultured en vitro for gene analysis.

These specific characteristics within the patient's genes are then compared in relationship with how--if at all--the various chemotherapy agents interact with these markers. This way lab technicians determine which of the 12 specific drugs families and 60 supplements work best, if any. In "hormone-driven" cancers the test identifies the best agents for effectively blocking hormonal action.

Upon completing this thorough analysis the Greek laboratory sends results to me. Then, after carefully reviewing this vital data, I construct a protocol involving a unique effective formula that marries the two most effective conventional drugs with all the best supplements. Once a patient agrees to pursue such a strategy, I often combine natural remedies and low-dose chemo to "work smart, rather than merely working hard."

Mainstream Oncologists Destroy the Body

The vast majority of advanced Stage IV cancer patients who visit conventional clinics are merely being poisoned by chemo that fails to do anything to eliminate their cancer. High-dose chemo often causes:

Chemo-brain syndrome: Commonly called "post-chemotherapy cognitive impairment," this hampers or wrecks the patient's cognitive abilities. According to the "Journal of Clinical Oncology," from 20 percent to 30 percent of people who undergo chemotherapy experience at least some form of chemo-brain syndrome. These outcomes have been so disturbing that the Journal of the National Cancer Institute has designated the condition as a real, measurable side effect. Some cancer survivors complain of a degradation of their cognitive abilities, plus decreases in their fluency and memory.

Cardiac toxicities: Sometimes called "cardiotoxicity," this condition occurs when the heart muscle sustains damage or the organ's ejection fraction reduces. These adverse characteristics, in turn, weaken the heart--which fails to adequately pump. The blood circulates with less efficiency than the organ had previously managed to accomplish consistently prior to the chemotherapy treatments. This can be measured by testing the ejection fraction (EF), which should be above 55 percent.

Peripheral neuropathies: This dreaded condition occurs when the body's sensory nerves become damaged or diseased. The numerous adverse symptoms that vary among patients can include the impairment of peripheral nerve organs, plus a hampered ability of movement and a decrease or loss of sensation. A vast array of additional nerve-related damage sometimes occurs, depending on which portion of the body's nerves are effected.

Bone marrow suppression: Sometimes called "myelotoxicity," this adverse medical condition generates one or all of numerous highly adverse effects. Besides the potential loss of normal blood clotting, some patients experience a severe infections that result from a decrease in the white cells responsible for providing immunity. Just as destructive, another condition called "anemia" can severely hamper the essential life-giving ability of red blood cells to carry oxygen.

Generalized rashes: Often lasting from five to 20 days, or perhaps much longer, this condition can generate bothersome itchiness, bumps, cracked or blistered skin, debilitating pain, and a variety of other adverse conditions such as secondary infections due to cracks or blisters.

Death: Conventional oncologists typically prefer to avoid discussing this topic at length with patients, but there is no escaping the fact that the needless or reckless over-use of chemotherapy often results in unnecessary death. Quite predictably many patients suffer from some or even all of the previously mentioned symptoms triggered by chemo, before dying from severe levels of these adverse side effects. Most allopathic cancer doctors refrain from admitting this disturbing fact--many of their patients are killed by the highly toxic and poisonous chemo, rather than succumbing to the cancer itself.

Better Choices Available

As a licensed oncologist I'm required by law and by industry protocol to give each Stage IV cancer patient the option of having conventional high-dose chemo "treatments"--instances where such a strategy would be required of standard oncologists.

The vast majority of people with advanced-stage cancer

who visit my clinic freely choose to avoid high doses of dangerous drugs. These patients usually follow my recommendation of a low-dose insulin potentiated chemo regimen, coupled with effective natural remedies--as determined by genetic testing.

For these individuals, my clinic administers low-dose fractionated insulin-potentiated regimens often referred to as "IPT." This technique "tricks the cancers" into opening up certain biological receptors. This happens due to a cancer's enhanced supply of insulin receptors.

These attributes leave the cancer open to potentially effective attacks by apoptosis-producing natural Poly-MVA administered by my clinic's medical personnel. This tactic often works because cancers can only thrive on simple sugars.

As a result, the cancers often die or go into remission, robbing the disease of its ultimate goal of killing the patient.

Important Book Emerged

One of my many patients became so impressed with this process that she wrote a compelling book about her positive experience being treated at Century Wellness Clinic.

Las Vegas-based businesswoman Diana Warren chronicled her story in "Say No to Radiation and Conventional Chemo--Winning My Battle Against Stage II Breast Cancer."

Prior to visiting my office Warren had gone to numerous mainstream oncologists. All of those medical professionals had insisted that she endure high-dose chemo treatments and radiation therapy.

Brave, intelligent and charismatic, Warren refused to cave in to their dangerous medical procedures. Instead, she let common sense serve as her guide, while ignoring the reckless protocol of mainstream physicians.

Warren undertook an in-depth research regimen, eventually deciding to visit my Reno-based clinic 450 miles from Las Vegas. Then, at my urging, Warren decided to take the "Greek Test," the chemosensitivity analysis.

The test results arrived within several weeks. Right away I worked with Warren in developing her personalized treatment regimen. We used a combination of the medications and supplements that the analysis had identified as the most effective for her body and particular type of cancer.

Warren's unique and specialized low-dose chemo treatment regimen began within several weeks at Century Wellness Clinic. Her cancer went into remission soon afterward, and at the time of this book's publication she had remained in remission for more than four years.

Numerous Positive Outcomes

Although I would never refer to myself in such glowing terms, numerous doctors and industry observers refer to me as a "virtual rock star within the medical industry."

Rooms filled with Homeopaths and their assistants often erupt into applause or give standing ovations as soon as I enter some medical industry conferences.

Always in high demand to attend such functions, I usually visit from six to 10 medical industry seminars yearly throughout the United States. You see, I continually learn more about fighting cancer while always developing effective, natural ways to fight the disease.

The positive focus on me and my clinic's techniques intensified when an intelligent and highly respected celebrity, Suzanne Somers, mentioned these critical details in worldwide media forums. Somers became so impressed that she described my clinic's cancer treatment procedures in her runaway 2010 bestseller, "Knockout: Interviews With Doctors Who are Curing Cancer--And How to Prevent Getting It in the First Place."

Huge percentages of my patients learn of Century Wellness Clinic via positive word-of-mouth from other people previously treated at my clinic. Streams of my patients first learn about me in Somers' book, or from the many books that I have written, or co-authored, or from publications where other writers praise my medical procedures.

Groundbreaking Doctor Pushes the Proverbial Envelope

An internationally acclaimed Los Angeles physician and surgeon, Doctor Patrick Soon-Shiong, has generally been using the same overall type of genomic-related testing and cancer treatment that my Century Wellness Clinic has been using with much success.

With an estimated personal worth of $11 billion, Soon-Shiong has been called "a genius, a showman, an innovator and a hypster," CBS News correspondent Doctor Sanjay Gupta, said in a "60 Minutes" program segment first aired on Dec. 7, 2014.

Like me, Soon-Shiong has had his advance-stage cancer treatment methodology come into question from some mainstream doctors. Those physicians insist that more time is needed to determine if such genomic testing and IPT treatments are effective and worthy of being recommended.

Yet as if echoing statements that I have made for more than 10 years, Soon-Shiong told Gupta that patients suffering from advance-stage cancer lack the luxury of time needed to wait for extensive testing and federal approval of new treatments.

"I'm incredibly encouraged to say that we are on the path," Soon-Shiong told "60 Minutes." "And the technology to do these things is not just hypothetical."

Soon-Shiong insists that scientists are learning to unmask cancer's molecular secrets, thanks largely to advances in DNA technology, coupled with a high-speed genome sequencing machine that he developed.

Similar to a process that I implemented at my clinic, the billionaire doctor prefers to have his advance-stage cancer patients undergo genomic testing. Like me, he strives to determine which specific drugs have the greatest probability of effectively killing the cancer of each patient.

Another similarity to my clinic's general protocol emerges from the fact that Soon-Shiong prefers administering low-dose chemo treatments.

Similar Overall Techniques Generate Success

In yet another significant similarity, Soon-Shiong insists that many people have a mistaken belief that cancer cells merely "grow." Instead, because of a mysterious and still-understood genetic mutation, the worst cancers essentially have *the inability to die*.

In our separate, unaffiliated medical practices while still employing similar overall strategies, Soon-Shiong's clinic and mine share a mutual professional and highly focused obsession with using genomic technology to determine the characteristics of cancer's strange mutation.

Ultimately, this often results in an improved long-term survival rate, always starting with a thorough analysis of each individual patient's genomic structure and specific type of cancer.

In best-case scenarios, these advances in cancer diagnosis and treatment ultimately lead to instances where the disease becomes categorized as completely gone or when cancer evolves into a "chronic health conditions" rather than fatal.

"Overall, these advancements are clicking into gear at a far greater pace than many people realize," I sometimes tell patients. "The old way of treating cancer patients with high-dose chemo should quickly emerge as 'a thing of the past,' replaced by a much more effective era."

2
Century Wellness Clinic Leads the Way

Almost every day the whole world seems to be banging on my clinic's door, eager and desperate to benefit from substantial advances in genomic technology.

Yet amazingly only an infinitesimal fraction of the 7 billion living people worldwide knows that my clinic uses these amazing anti-cancer techniques.

My office doors are always open weekdays, except on a handful of U.S. holidays and during the brief span from Christmas through New Year's Day.

As you might very well imagine, my office phones are continually "ringing off the hook" while people ask for appointments.

Many patients tell me that they're pleased and delighted upon discovering that my staff is eager to answer any questions that they might have.

Demand Continues to Intensify

The patient load at Century Wellness Clinic continues on a steady increase. Every step of the way we strive to make the process as stress-free and easy as possible for each person eager for an examination and treatment.

I' have already stated the following in the first chapter, but I need to re-emphasize the details here because the important facts are essential to all my patients:

Many people visiting for the first time admit they're impressed by the fact that nearly two-thirds of my Stage IV cancer patients remain alive and in remission from the disease--4.5 years after their initial treatments at Century Wellness Clinic.

Remember, this means that six out of every 10 worst-stage cancer patients that I treat remain alive, most relatively healthy and capable of enjoying life to the fullest.

By contrast, according to numerous nationwide medical reports, only two out of every 100 Stage IV cancer patients survive when treated by mainstream oncologists.

So, knowing these details, who would you choose--the doctors required to administer high-dose poison in all such cases, or me, an expert at administering an effective combination of low-dose chemo, natural remedies and healthy supplements?

Take These Important Steps

To help optimize results and make their excursions as stress-free as possible, all first-time patients visiting Century Wellness Clinic can:

Call: 775-827-0707, or toll free 877-789-0707; tell the receptionist your health situation, so that we can start the process of potentially making a reservation.

Records: Upon making a reservation, you must bring copies of your records from your current doctor, or send us that information before arriving. This information should include any and all available reports regarding oncology, pathology, surgery, chemotherapy, X-rays, scans, laboratory tests, narrative summaries, and a list of all medications and supplements.

Frailty: Like all doctors, we generally are unable to treat patients who have become "extremely frail;" under this condition the person's body mass and weight have dropped to precipitously low levels--while muscles have nearly disappeared.

Prior Treatments: Preferably before their first visit to Century Wellness, patients should avoid being treated elsewhere by mainstream oncologists. The high-dose chemo and radiation administered by those doctors seriously weakens and damages the body--thereby decreasing the potential effectiveness of subsequent treatments. Homeopaths refer to people with cancer who refrain from chemo and radiation prior to visiting doctors of natural medicine as "virginal treatment patients." Although we prefer treating "virginal patients," in many instances my clinic accepts people with cancer who already have been treated by

24

conventional oncologists. In order to be accepted, such candidates must communicate with a member of my staff before a decision is made.

Travel & Accommodations: New and returning patients make their own arrangements for travel and lodging. The Reno area has numerous high-quality hotels and restaurants at mid-range and high-end prices. Car rentals via Reno-Tahoe International Airport are available for those who travel by air, and shuttle services are provided by most major hotel-casinos in the region.

Location: Century Wellness Clinic is at 521 Hammill Lane in South Reno, an ideal site just one block from on-ramps and off-ramps to U.S. Interstate 580--one of the region's two primary highways. A north-south arterial, I-580 provides easy access to the airport, all of the region's primary hotels, and the region's primary east-west highway, U.S. Interstate 80. Travel time to or from the airport and the clinic is about 10 minutes.

Activities: During "free" time when not undergoing medical examinations or treatments, patients, their relatives or friends have a vast array of options for fun, relaxing, energizing or restful activities. The high-desert region surrounding Reno, which is at 4,500 feet above sea level, has hundreds of miles of hiking trails providing panoramic views. The city is just a one-hour drive from Lake Tahoe, an ideal summer playground. Nestled in the Sierra at 6,200 feet above sea level, as North America's largest alpine lake, Tahoe has easy access to dozens of ski resorts popular during winter. Just as enticing, the historic Comstock Lode mining town of Virginia City, where the legendary writer Mark Twain began his journalism career for the "Territorial Enterprise" in the 1860s, is just a 30-minute drive southeast of Reno. Virginia City has numerous popular attractions including museums, and historic saloons such as the the world famous Bucket of Blood saloon.

Expected stays: Patients visiting for initial examinations and chemosensitivity testing usually stay from several days to one week. Those undergoing treatment regimens of low-dose chemo, effective natural remedies and supplements usually stay from two to three weeks. Subsequent visits for standard examinations are usually recommended for patients who have undergone treatments, so that I can monitor each person's progress in beating cancer. Follow-up visits for examinations usually are arranged in three- or six-month, or one-year intervals; these spans hinge on the type of cancer a patient had, the current suspected severity of the disease; and whether the cancer has gone into--or seems to progressing into--remission.

Additional treatment: Some patients occasionally require or request follow-up treatment regimens if their cancer remains active following the initial round.

Various ailments: Century Wellness Clinic treats patients suffering from many types of ailments, particularly cancer. We treat all types of the disease in any bodily area and at every level of severity; besides advanced Stage IV cancer, the clinic treats patients suffering from less severe levels including Stage II and Stage III. Patients need to know that unless effectively treated all types of cancer can worsen to the dreaded Stage IV; the worst-stage cancers invariably lead to death unless successfully treated. In addition, many patients learn prior to their initial visits to Century Wellness that mainstream oncologists strive to administer poisonous and deadly high-dose chemo to patients suffering from the less severe Stage II or Stage III levels of the disease--not just Stage IV.

Critical Patient Choices

Keep in mind that as previously stated, throughout every phase of each patient's examinations and treatment I give the patient the option of making critical choices.

This marks a sharp contrast from the style of mainstream oncologists, who essentially say without using such specific words: "It's my way, or the highway."

I give each patient the option of receiving natural remedies that are proven highly effective, always with the patient's physical and mental well-being in mind.

In doing so, I'm essentially following the philosophy of Doctor Benjamin Rush, a signer of the Declaration of Independence and the personal physician of U.S. President George Washington.

"Unless we put medical freedom into the Constitution, the time will come when medicine will organize into an undercover dictatorship," said Rush, a founding father of the United States who died in 1813 at age 67. "To restrict the art of healing to one class of men and deny equal privileges to others will cause a Bastille of medical science.

"All such laws are un-American and despotic, and have no place in a republic. The Constitution of this republic should make a special privilege for medical freedom."

To the detriment of all types of patients, no such provisions were included in the USA's founding documents. Since then mainstream doctors have run roughshod over patients' rights; these physicians have used their political allies to implement and control federal agencies that require or sanction the use of ineffective, costly, and poisonous deadly drugs.

Whole Body and Soul

Effectively treating patients can only happen when addressing the whole body, the mind and what I sometimes call the person's "positive spirit or soul."

Unlike mainstream oncologists who poison the entire body in an effort "to fix an isolated cancer," I incorporate a whole-body strategy using mostly natural remedies.

Besides administering low-dose chemo with natural remedies, personnel at my clinic also help address numerous issues in order to improve each patient's overall health. Among these critical health-enhancing tactics that mainstream oncologists ignore are:

Balance: We show each patient how to achieve a balanced lifestyle using an ideal combination of rest, exercise, sleep, nutrition and activities suited for emotional harmony.

Detoxify: Clean the body of foreign or unnatural substances that are likely to damage overall health, while sometimes also sometimes triggering cancer.

Diet: The common saying that "you are what you eat" remains true, sometimes leading to cancer due to unhealthy diets. So, we teach patients about good nutrition.

Empower: As previously stated, we give each patient choices about treatment, recovery and strategies to achieve or to maintain optimal health.

Information: We teach patients the critical details that they must know to detect, prevent and control cancer.

Sugar: We teach each patient that common sugars, particular when ingested in high amounts, are a leading cause of cancer--which "love and thrives" on this substance.

Supplements: Use the supplements identified by chemosensitivity testing as the most helpful for a specific cancer patient; these products contain vitamins, minerals and various herbs. They serve as the backbone for good overall physical, mental and spiritual health.

Target Specific Cancers

I have developed unique, individualized strategies to effectively battle each form of cancer.

This is unlike mainstream oncologists who--as previously stated--use an ill-advised and ineffective "one-size-fits-all" approach to almost every form of the disease.

By analyzing an individual's chemosensitivity test, physical examination and medical records, I'm able to marry the best natural remedies in combination with low-dose chemo, along with supplements identified as the most effective for the person.

Doctors classify each form of cancer based on the bodily area where the disease started. Compounding the challenge, each type of cancer has a unique growth rate, pattern of spreading and response to specific treatments.

Many physicians and particularly Homeopaths have

deemed me as perhaps the world's premiere expert at developing and matching the ideal and most effective treatment for each type of cancer.

Chemosensitivity tests are particularly helpful because each person has a unique, one-of-a-kind genomic structure unlike any other person.

Risk Factors Play a Role

Intense and continuous worldwide genomic research has been identifying and confirming what many physicians have suspected for a long time.

Genomic research has confirmed that some individuals have a greater likelihood than the general population of developing specific types of cancer.

For instance, women from some families have a far greater chance of developing breast cancer than most females throughout the general population.

At least some good news has emerged. Scientists have confirmed that the inherited probability of cancer is less prevalent than previously thought.

As a result, some researchers and medical facilities have informally categorized most cancer causes as instances where the individual is a victim of "bad luck."

Many severe risk factors sharply increase the probability of getting cancer. Besides smoking or chewing tobacco, these include exposure to chemicals, ultraviolet light, free radicals in foods, red or processed meats, sugar, air pollution and many more.

In addition, each specific risk factor increases a person's chances of getting certain cancers. For instance, smoking or chewing tobacco sharply increases a person's risk of developing cancers of the lung, tongue, mouth, larynx, and other organs. Scientists blame most skin cancers on excessive exposure to the sun or suntanning machines.

Most tumors are benign or lacking cancer; such tumors are usually non-threatening, except in rare exceptions.

In all instances of cancer, a person's chances of "being cured" increase drastically the sooner the disease is discovered and treated; cancers that are allowed to grow and spread over extended periods without being treated sharply increase the chances of developing into deadly advanced Stage IV levels of the disease.

My "War Plan" in Fighting Cancer

In the fight against cancer, patients at Century Wellness Clinic might think of me as a proverbial five-star general or a commander-in-chief.

Under my continual command the clinic's staff administers at least 17 strategies, many that I have personally designed to destroy cancer. With added importance, some of these strategies strive to put each patient on a pathway toward optimal overall health.

Besides the unique chemosensitivity testing of whole blood, one of these key techniques briefly mentioned earlier involves the low-dose fractionated regimens sometimes called "IPT."

As previously stated, when using a unique system that I personally developed, the process strives to "trick" or "fool" the disease into opening certain receptors within the cancer's cells. This happens in part because cancers desperately crave energy-producing sugar and oxygen.

I work to ensure that this natural process opens biological receptors. When this happens the cancer is left wide-open to horrific attacks, while the rest of the body remains unharmed and safe.

The typical weaponry that I employ here involves a natural substance, the harmless and effective Poly-MVA expertly administered by my staff. This is usually done on alternate days with low-dose fractionated chemotherapy, levels much smaller and far less harmful to the body than chemo typically administered by mainstream oncologists.

Napoleonic Battles Against Cancer

Although despotic, often cruel and heartless, the famed French Emperor and General Napoléon Bonaparte of the early 19th Century remains world-famous for his dastardly war tactics of suddenly attacking enemies using extreme unconventional tactics.

At least within the realm of battling cancer, many of my patients think of me as using "Napoleonic battle plans against the disease within the practices of both oncology and Homeopathy."

Highly detailed books could be separately written and published about each of my most popular and effective cancer-fighting strategies. Besides chemosensitivity tests, IPT, and low-dose fractionated chemotherapy, here is a brief summary of some of the most effective methods frequently used at Century Wellness Clinic:

Healthful water: Because healthful, pure water can boost energy while ridding the body of harmful and potentially cancerous impurities, we provide patients with access to pH 9.0 "alkaline H2O pH therapy." The water is at an optimal alkaline level, the opposite from the harmful acidic range. This strategy serves an important role because cancer thrives within an acidic environment; the pH levels of most cancer patients are typically far more acidic than alkaline.

Nutritional guidance: What a person chooses to eat plays a critical role in either generating or preventing cancer. Many of these "poor" and "good" choices hinge on whether a particular food is within the healthful alkaline or unhealthy acidic ranges. We show patients meal plans developed for their unique personal situations. These details can be found in my hot-selling book, the "Forsythe Anti-Cancer Diet;" it's available in paper or e-reader form via all major bookstores and online eBook venues.

Individualized nutrition: Besides the advice on diet briefly mentioned above, we develop cancer-fighting and cancer-preventing regimens that include specific foods, vitamins, and herbs. As I often tell patients, natural substances such as these generally are far more preferable than unnatural or synthetic drugs typically administered by mainstream oncologists. Besides helping to boost overall health, such products serve as just one of the many ways that we help give the body a fighting, natural chance against cancer.

Immune Enhancement: Cancer typically compromises or weakens the body's immune system, often robbing the person of energy and the ability to fight the disease. To counteract this detrimental condition, we administer a Vitamin-C high-dose immune booster that patients receive intravenously as a standard procedure. Often loaded with vital additional vitamins and supplements, these immune-enhancing sessions often sharply increase the body's natural ability to battle certain ailments--particularly cancer. Besides cancer patients, my clinic treats people with other health issues that compromise or weaken immunity.

Biological Response Modifiers: Besides the immune enhancement technique listed immediately above, we also employ "biological response modifiers" that are sometimes called "BRMs." Remember that as mentioned earlier, the effective strategies that I employ typically strive to kill at least 90 percent of a patient's cancer, and from that point the person's immune system plays a critical role in fighting and successfully killing the remainder of the disease. Similar to substances naturally produced by the body and often created by scientists in laboratories, BRMs super-charge the body's natural response to infection and to cancer. This "immunotherapy" treatment process enhances the body's immune systems, particularly natural defenses against cancer. Also, because my clinic serves patients with ailments other than cancer, we sometimes use BRMs to affectively address such adverse conditions as rheumatoid arthritis. Although comprised of natural substances, the administering of BRMs on extremely rare occasion generates adverse symptoms such as diarrhea, nausea, vomiting and loss of appetite. Thus, BRMs should only be taken in a professional medical environment that monitors patients.

Bio-Oxidative Therapy: A super-powerful tool among

natural healing methods, the natural process called "bio-oxidative therapy" serves as a stong anti-oxidant and cancer killer. One of only a small percentage of physicians to use this strategy, I have learned first-hand many times that bio-oxidative therapy robs cancer of low oxygen that the disease needs to live, grow and thrive. Unlike humans and all mammals, cancer gets its oxygen from the fermentation process, rather than breathing from the environment. At my recommendation and upon patient approval, I use bio-oxidative therapy to surround cancer cells with oxygen. This high-oxygen environment can significantly decrease the disease's ability to grow and to divide. Meantime, this therapy typically stimulates receptors in white blood cells, thus boosting the immune system and fortifying the body's natural strength and effectiveness in attacking cancer. Perhaps just as impressive, this therapy increases the body's natural production of interferon, interleukin-2 and tumor necrosis factor--all factors that sharply boost the body's natural cancer fighting processes. Meantime, bio-oxidative therapy also often improves the health of patients who have been ill, thanks to the ability of this process to increase oxygen tension in bodily tissues.

Lifestyle guidance: Clinic staff members often teach or suggest ways for an individual patient to enjoy life to the fullest extent possible. Such positive behavioral changes often make the person feel better both physically and emotionally, thereby decreasing the likelihood that a cancer will worsen or return. When giving this advice, my personnel consider numerous simultaneous factors including the person's type and severity of cancer, level of remission, overall health, and all other ailments currently experienced by the individual.

Professional referrals: As a highly experienced doctor with extensive medical industry contacts throughout Northern Nevada and worldwide, I sometimes refer patients who need additional services to other medical professionals ranging from surgeons to radiologists.

Second opinions: After initially receiving the diagnosis of physicians elsewhere, some people visit Century Wellness Clinic to seek a "second opinion" from me or other doctors on my staff. Sometimes we reach similar conclusions, although in numerous instances either I or my personnel generate findings that differ from what the patient had been told elsewhere.

Coping skills: Century Wellness Clinic offers individual and group counseling, unlike the vast majority of mainstream oncologists and cancer treatment facilities nationwide. At my clinic, skilled advisers highly knowledgeable in medicine and optimal lifestyles teach patients or their families how to cope and excel in key issues. Patients and their families learn optimal ways to administer effective healthcare, plus suggested methods on handling daily lifestyle tasks or personal responsibilities.

Patients Deserve Priority Status

At Century Wellness Clinic, every patient gets "priority status;" they all deserve and receive respect without being ignored or told, "Do this and do that. Take this poison, because you have no other choice."

The doctors and personnel at my facility strongly embrace this highly coveted mission statement. We strive to show each patient that the clinic truly cares, while effectively working in an effort to achieve the best possible results.

Blessed with a keen knowledge of the art and science of medicine, I continually draw upon all treatment modalities ranging from the most advanced conventional therapies to mainstream medicine. All along, I also incorporate the most effective remedies of Homeopathic medicine, primarily natural therapies ignored by mainstream oncologists.

Using these medical systems as a solid foundation for giving all patients the best possible care, I have developed four options uniquely designed to fulfill their desires:

One: Fractionated conventional chemotherapy alone

Two: Fractional chemotherapy, plus Homeopathic treatments including Insulin Potentiated Therapy (IPT) Lite (TM).

Three: Complimentary Homeopathic and/or naturopathic modalities alone

Four: Best supportive therapy

Based on my intensive studies, I have discovered that superior results occur when using combination treatments of: IPT with fractionated (low-dose) chemotherapy; Homeopathic intravenous remedies; and immune-stimulating supplements including organic herbs.

Along with my staff throughout the course of treating thousands of patients, I have developed intense studies on: Paw-Paw, a naturally grown substance deemed highly effective in cancer treatment; Poly-MVA, a uniquely formulated combination of minerals and amino acids designed to support cellular energy and promote overall good health, while also highly effective for treating cancer; the Forsythe Immune Protocol, a highly effective immune-enhancing process that I personally developed to significantly boost positive results in the treatment of my cancer patients; and a combination of the Forsythe Immune Protocol, CST and IPT--which means chemosensitivity testing, followed by IPT.

A "Bill of Rights" for Patients

Determined to counteract the "dogmatic rules" imposed by mainstream oncologists who refuse to allow patients to make vital choices regarding their own health, I have developed an essential "Bill of Rights" that all people with cancer can embrace. Among some of the most important proclamations:

Positive attitude: Each patient has a right to refrain from becoming afraid or discouraged, always cognizant that at various times in recent years medical literature has chronicled cures for all types of cancer.

Alternative path: Patients have a right to chose a unique, extremely rare integrative medical oncologist such as me because I'm highly skilled at treating their entire bodies with harmless and effective natural remedies--plus drugs when necessary.

High-dose chemo: Patients have a right to refuse extensive high-dose chemo regimens that mainstream oncologists insist on administering. When and if such a refusal is made, the patient should have a right to seek out the services of an extremely rare integrative medical oncologist such as me--capable of administering effective natural remedies.

Remain skeptical: Patients have a right to "keep an open mind about issues," while also remaining skeptical when reading or hearing about the supposed results of various clinical studies--particularly instances where two or more drugs are used.

Show spunk: Each patient has a right to peacefully "stand his or her own ground" as a self-preservation measure. Such instances might involve politely leaving an oncologist's office when the doctor mentions "hospice care" or "getting your affairs in order." Such statements indicate that the physician has given up on you; all patients have a right to embrace an attitude that: "I will never give up on myself."

Food choices: Patients have a right and a responsibility to themselves to adopt good eating habits, following the advice of their Homeopaths, physicians and dietitians.

Avoid unnecessary tests: Patients have a right to refuse over-testing, particularly procedures that involve radiation; radiological scans that target various areas of the body's overall immune system are particularly dangerous. Such procedures endanger overall health, increasing the likelihood that immune defenses will fail to work at optimal levels.

Alternative medicines: Patients have a right to know about, to use and to benefit from effective natural remedies that mainstream oncologists refuse to mention or to use. Of particular importances are beneficial supplements that often emerge as extremely helpful and essential in fighting cancer; supplements also eliminate carcinogens and toxins from the body.

Beware of media: Patients have a right and a responsibility to themselves to remain wary of advertisements or promotions that strive to fool them. For instance, some cancer centers claim to have the latest "pinpointed radiology procedures."

Refuse certain surgeries: Particularly among those with advanced Stage IV cancer, patients have a right to avoid a doctor's insistence that they undergo aggressive surgical procedures. These include second-look operations and devastating head-and-neck surgeries requiring tracheotomy and/or gastric feeding tubes.

Limit drugs: Patients have a right to limit the amount of drugs that they take. Whenever possible a patient should be able to take the smallest number of drugs, administered at the lowest-possible doses needed to fight their cancer. This strategy can minimize or prevent the destruction of the person's vital immune system.

Patients Praise Me

I receive heart-felt, compelling and emotional letters or emails each week from all over the world, sent by patients extremely grateful for their improved health.

"I'm so grateful to remain alive," is a phrase signifying a common theme. "I'm eternally grateful for the new lease on life that you have given me."

Some of my now-healthy former patients retell their stories, recounting the fact that they had previously been told elsewhere that: "You are going to die."

Imagine being informed that you are definitely going to be killed within a certain limited number of weeks or months, only to subsequently learn after finally being treated by me that you are going to live.

While glad to receive these messages, I refrain from dwelling on them--partly due to the need to continually concentrate on my job of "saving" as many people as possible.

Of course, not all of my patients survive. Yet as previously stated, the five-year survival rate of my advanced Stage IV cancer patients is far greater than the national average. Remember, according to my clinic's current study involving 850 patients, only two out of every 100 Stage IV cancer patients treated by mainstream oncologists survive, while 67 of such people that I treat remain alive at five years.

Essential Details

As previously mentioned, even following my success in treating cancer patients, I never can, have or will issue any guarantee that any patient will be cured or experience a significant improvement in his or her overall medical condition.

With this clearly understood, readers should remain fully cognizant of the fact that the details that I have provided in this book are strictly for educational and informational purposes only.

In addition, you should refrain from considering any or all statements that I have made here as medical advice--specifically because at this point we can assume that you are not yet a patient of mine.

I only make specific diagnosis and issue recommendations individually to each of my patients after conducting a thorough physical examination and reviewing medical records.

With these "disclaimer" factors clearly understood, my clinic welcomes inquiries from potential patients. Also, prospective patients should know that Century Wellness Clinic is an out-patient facility without overnight accommodations.

3
Dangerous Process Revealed

I can proclaim without any reservation whatsoever that the FDA, allopathic physicians and oncologists are "dead wrong" when insisting that natural remedies "never work at all."

Most unwilling to believe the FDA's destructive propaganda, my patients have every right to discover for themselves that "natural remedies are far safer and much more effective overall than unnatural drugs--much more preferred."

Many of these patients essentially tell themselves that "I would rather give myself a fighting chance, than subject my body to worthless poisons that undoubtedly would kill me."

Indeed, I have learned first-hand many times that natural remedies usually "work just as good as or far better than synthetic or unnatural pharmaceutical products."

As an integrative oncologist, I am licensed to administer drugs including chemotherapy made by Big Pharma. Meantime, as a Homeopath I also can prescribe natural, effective and harmless remedies that mainstream doctors avoid, and which they are prohibited by law from providing.

Consider My Expertise
Bowing to the requests of consumers and medical experts who look to me for guidance, I have written more than 20 hot-selling books and chapters geared to teach common consumers how to maintain good health using natural remedies proven as effective.

Sure enough, results from my own patients--and from numerous scientific studies as well--prove beyond any reasonable doubt that substances from Mother Nature cure or relieve symptoms from a variety of ailments. This happens without adverse side effects.

To say or even to imply that synthetic drugs should be used

for all ailments is a blatant and reckless disservice to consumers everywhere.

The general public deserves and has a right to much better remedies and services than those provided by Big Pharma and the mainstream medical industry.

Exciting Revelations

I began working as a mainstream oncologist in the early 1970s. From then through the mid-1990s I treated more than 10,000 cancer patients.

In keeping with nationwide trends, only about 2 percent of my patients suffering from advanced Stage IV cancer survived through that period. During that span, I administered dangerous and usually deadly chemotherapy to these individuals--in keeping with protocol required by the standard allopathic medical industry.

As you might imagine, this frustrated and saddened me. During that span, so many of my patients died that if buried en masse in a single community their corpses could have filled an entire graveyard. The fact that I was competent and "did everything possible" under medical industry guidelines failed to make any difference in patient outcomes.

After learning about the benefits of natural medicine, starting in the mid-1990s I did what only a handful of oncologists have ever dared. While maintaining my busy medical practice, I attended college during my 50s in order to become a licensed Homeopath while maintaining a standard medical license.

Some people might have complained that I had essentially turned my back on mainstream medicine, but nothing was further from the truth.

Life Springs from Nature

From the mid-1990s through the initial decade of the 21st Century I worked non-stop in developing effective treatments, as described fully in many of my books including "Take Control of Your Cancer," and the "Forsythe Anti-Cancer Diet."

As previously indicated, various natural substances play an essential role in generating a current 67-percent Stage IV cancer survival rate at my clinic--thanks largely to the significant advancements in genomics during the past two decades.

Much of this became possible thanks largely to the intense research by practitioners of natural medicines. These "doctors or community medical experts" have lived in many societies worldwide for thousands of years.

Rather than relying solely on dangerous synthetic drugs, most cultures across Europe, Asia, Africa, South America and Central America readily accept and appreciate the effectiveness of natural remedies.

Threatening Their Monopoly

A dangerous and corrupt link or economic bond is seemingly unbreakable between mainstream physicians and the major drug manufacturers.

This unholy alliance stems largely from the fact that Big Pharma depends on doctors for its survival. Without doctors on their side the countless billions of dollars generated yearly by drug manufacturers would be impossible.

Without question, standard mainstream allopathic doctors in the United States are collectively the biggest organized "drug-pushing organization in world history"--all with the blessing of our national government.

Perhaps just as destructive, although they avoid telling you so, as an overall profession standard allopathic doctors depend on Big Pharma for major perks ranging from free lunches and revenue sharing to expense-paid vacations.

All a doctor needs to do to qualify for these grab-bags of goodies is merely to prescribe as many doses as possible of a specific pharmaceutical product. Shockingly, this happens on a consistent, regular and predictable daily basis, even in specific instances where these harmful, addictive and expensive substances are unnecessary.

Tragically, many doctors who engage in such tactics on an extreme scale are violating the Hippocratic Oath of ethical medical industry standards.

Positive Action Becomes Critical

The many diverse yet interlinking issues serve as the basis for my strong desire to educate the public about treatments that eventually will be generated via genomics research.

Without exaggeration, as previously indicated these various compelling topics are likely to impact people everwhere throughout the remaining course of mankind.

Indeed, decisions that society makes during the early 21st Century regarding treatments generated from genomics research will have a profound impact for many thousands of years. Many issues have emerged, including:

Health: Rather than relying on synthetic drugs, will society demand natural remedies stemming from genetics research whenever possible in order to avoid adverse side effects?

Availability: Will recommended treatments for specific ailments be widely available to the general public, or provided only to a "select few?"

Costs: What, if anything, will be done to limit the costs of the specific treatments, curtailing excessive and unwarranted Big Pharma profits?

Bureaucracy: What input will the general public be allowed to give on a genuine basis, while the criteria and infrastructure of this upgraded medical industry is launched?

Homeopaths: What assurances, if any, will the public have that Homeopaths are given a key role in generating recommended treatments based on data from genetic research?

Target Critical Issues

Cognizant of these critical issues, scientists and doctors worldwide need to take decisive action within the next several years. Physicians must ensure that the infrastructures of these various projects guarantee that natural remedies will receive continual consideration. Otherwise the quality of health care services would fail to reach its greatest potential, namely the development and use of harmless, inexpensive and effective natural remedies--rather than merely relying on synthetic drugs.

Mindful of the critical importance of this issue, those of us medical professionals aware of the importance of Homeopathy and Naturopathy need to do a better job educating the general public about these specific challenges.

Meantime, an overriding danger looms that numerous less-than-optimal drugs will be "set in stone as required via protocols," genomics-generated treatment systems developed by mainstream medicine due to its nefarious ties with Big Pharma.

So, a serious question arises: Could there be a danger that technology developed by mainstream doctors, organizations and researchers tied to Big Pharma might result in requirements mandating the use of dangerous drugs?

An understandable fear emerges here. You see, when and if such "apparent" advancements are made without scientists making any effort to pinpoint natural remedies, consumers would be given only one option from mainstream medicine: "Take these unnatural, expensive and dangerous drugs although you might not need or want them."

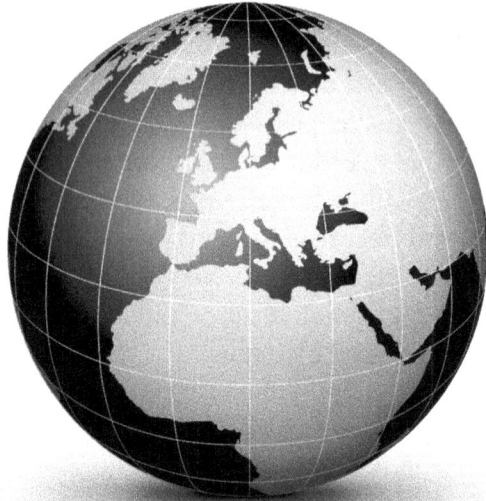

Imagine a world where doctors cure cancer
within days, senior citizens enjoy bodies that
seemingly refuse to age, and most crippling
diseases disappear.
Just as exciting within this fantastic
new realm, scientists replicate DNA to produce
the smartest, healthiest, most resilient and
super-creative human beings.

4
Milestone Medical Advancements

Rapid-fire advancements keep improving medical care worldwide, leading to potential cures for many diseases thanks to massive international genomic research programs.

Often misunderstood by the general public, the Human Genome Project already has led to huge advancements in fighting everything from cancer to Alzheimer's disease.

All this became possible when scientists mapped out human life's once-secret genomic code from the early 1990s until 2003.

Since then, finally armed with the proverbial "map of all life" for the first time in history, scientists have remained diligent using the data for launching many genomic research projects needed to develop cures.

The effort has become so all-encompassing and important that advances in modern medicine through the 2020s likely will benefit humanity for thousands of years.

Fantastic Possibilities Abound

Imagine a world where doctors cure cancer within days, senior citizens enjoy bodies that seemingly refuse to age, and most crippling diseases disappear.

Just as exciting within this fantastic new realm, scientists replicate DNA to produce the smartest, healthiest, most resilient and super-creative human beings.

Ideally, at least if some scientists are to be believed, sideline research into the universal genomic code also could be used to end famine.

Yes, envision a world where scientists modify the DNA within crops to produce fast-growing, safe, tasty and nutritious foods.

If all goes well with these overall efforts, the many benefits from genetics research could help ensure the long-term survival of the human species.

Exciting Future

In a best-case scenario, what had once been the so-called "laws of nature" essentially will get "turned upside down" for good.

If all goes as hoped, these advancements will have far greater impact than when explorers more than 500 years ago proved that the world is oval rather than flat.

The age-old saying that "only two things are guaranteed in life--death and taxes" could become a thing from the past. Many people would seemingly never die, a distinct possibility.

Under ideal conditions, the vast majority of humans would never suffer from today's common and debilitating conditions ranging from obesity to diabetes.

Just as essential, thanks to genomic research into the human brain, the overall intelligence of people throughout society would increase far higher than today.

Prepare for the Near-Future

Some of these substantial advancements are likely to occur far sooner than many people realize, unaware such efforts are underway.

Assuming that such progress continues, people born since the dawn of the 21st Century are likely to enjoy far healthier lives as adults than those of us born in the 1900s.

Wide-eyed optimists predict these upcoming advancements will emerge as a significant boost to many economic sectors, from food production to educational institutions and much more.

Some casual observers seem to view these scenarios as fantasy, while scientists involved in the research consider such strides as "just around the corner."

Many of these technological advancements are likely to

click into gear at a steady pace, far too complex for many people to understand.

Impact All Aspects of Life

Technological advancements stemming from the Human Genome Project should impact virtually all aspects of human life.

Rather than merely concentrating on the health benefits of individual people, scientists are using genomics to replicate the human brain in developing robots.

Far more impressive, experts also are using genomics technology to develop Artificial Intelligence--an effort that might eventually enable machines to "think and learn."

Upon first discovering news of these planned advancements many people understandably become either optimistic or apprehensive.

To say that many people will become "emotionally shocked" or at least surprised by such revelations would be far from an exaggeration.

Learn Essential Basics

With steadily increasing frequency in recent years, people from around the world have asked me to give my opinion on genomics--a subject that confuses many of them.

"Prepare for a vastly different world, considerable changes in all aspects of your life and the lives of everyone that you know," I tell patients who ask, many who have traveled to my West Coast U.S. medical office. "Discoveries in genomic science have become so significant that amazing new developments are announced almost daily."

From my view these individual and overall efforts can never be stopped, no matter how much we ever might want to try.

Perhaps because many doctors consider me one of the world's leading cancer physicians, streams of people have started asking me whether genomics can be used to eradicate the disease.

"Luckily, thanks to genomics advancements, that's already

happening--at least for many people when conditions are ideal," I say. "Right now, however, the only way to benefit from genomics is to visit a rare doctor like me, capable of--or with access to-- using that technology."

Accentuate the Positives

Rather than allowing ourselves to become confounded by the critical issues already mentioned, we all need to acknowledge and to appreciate that the Human Genome Project--and the many genomic research efforts that it inspired--hail among the most significant and beneficial scientific advancements in human history.

In summary, scientists have "unlocked the secret code."

Thanks to their efforts from 1990 until April 2003, doctors and researchers for the first time have the entire blueprint of the countless millions of genes in an individual person.

Think of this extraordinary finding as a proverbial roadmap. The intricate detail lists every highway, byway and road within the DNA structure of the human body.

To put this into focus, envision the first maps the explorers made of earth, from when Christopher Columbus landed in the Americas in 1492 and lasting through around 1700. Thanks to those efforts scientists and explorers finally had drawings or schematics of the globe.

Press Forward With Research

Modern scientists involved in the primary significant research efforts stemming from the Human Genome Project have been the equivalent of early researchers who studied geography in the 1700s and 1800s.

Although during the 1500s and 1600s scientists and geologists had developed a rather crude global map, in 1700 they still needed many more generations to accurately map the entire earth while incorporating details of each new-found culture.

Well, a somewhat similar challenge faces today's genomic

researchers, except in a much different and far more complex sense.

As previously stated, since 2003 scientists have had the entire map of the human genome sequence. Yet now in a critical research phase, they need to analyze and quantify each proverbial highway and byway in the human structure. Unless this is done with great focus and skill, merely having the overall map of a human being's genomic and DNA makeup would be of little use.

Human Genome Project leaders were right on track when they announced shortly after the 21st Century began that essentially their work had only just begun, although they had finished processing basics of the entire human genomic map.

Tremendous Infrastructure Needed

The chromosomes in an individual person range from about 50 million to 300 million base pairs, according to the Human Genome Research Institute, part of the U.S. National Institutes of Health.

With these significant figures in mind, imagine the complexity and formidable challenges facing researchers assigned with the task of identifying how or under what circumstances each pair zone effects or generates specific diseases or ailments.

The challenge becomes even more formidable upon adding to this the critical need to identify, analyze and improve upon specific remedies for each pairing problem.

As an overall group, doctors and scientists remain confident that they'll be able to accomplish this, leading to the previously mentioned significant medical advancements.

Yet the timetable for completing the essential follow-up research remains a "great unknown." Scientists seemed right on track in 2003 when they announced that the necessary follow-up research would last several decades at the very least.

Multiple Disciplines Required

Accomplishing the essential follow-up phases leading to

potential "cures" requires multiple disciplines working effectively in unison. In much the same way that an orchestra needs to practice in order to fine-tune and ultimately perfect a melody, those involved in a variety of significant genomic research efforts are "continually getting their act together."

Think of the following to put all this into clear perspective. An orchestra might have the world's greatest piano player, the most talented violinist and the best percussionist. But the musicians will fail to approach perfection when performing as a combined unit unless each player listens carefully to the others and continually modifies and improves efforts. Whatever their individual talent levels, all musicians need to practice together with the common goal of achieving an ideal sound. Musicians call this "the groove."

Well, genomics researchers need to accomplish their tasks by using a unique form of fine-tuning and practicing systems on a much grander scale.

For success to occur, leaders of the various interrelated genomics research projects need to effectively incorporate a vast array of scientific and professional disciplines. Among them:

Information technology: Use and employ computer experts to continually analyze massive quantities of information.

Mathematics: Experts within mathematics, and especially within the realm of physics, to calculate, analyze and quantify the continual inflow of critical information.

Biology: Experts in biology to analyze the data and conclusions amassed by IT and math experts, while also working with those team members to help fine-tune their process.

Medical teams: Highly trained experts who obtain biological specimens from patients, adhering to strict criteria for collecting samples.

Medical facilities: Cooperating hospitals, university research laboratories and doctors collect patients' data, then sent to core genomic research teams for analysis.

Major Technology Breakthroughs

The many current genomics research projects have become possible thanks to recent groundbreaking advancements in significant yet unrelated fields: computer technology and analysis; improved communication thanks to the Internet; and medical research techniques.

From among the many thousands of pages issued by the National Human Genome Research Institute, at least one document summarizes the massive task facing researchers as they continually strive to quantify and to analyze huge amounts of data.

"The primary method used by the HGP (Human Genome Project) (researchers) to produce the finished version of the human genetic code is map-based, or BAC-based, sequencing. BAC is the acronym for 'bacterial artificial chromosome.'" the report says. "Human DNA is fragmented into pieces that are relatively large but still manageable in size (between 150,000 and 200,000 base pairs).

"The fragments are cloned in bacteria, which store and replicate the human DNA so that it can be prepared in quantities large enough for sequencing. If carefully chosen to minimize overlap, it takes about 20,000 different BAC clones to contain the 3 billion pairs of bases of the human genome. A collection of BAC clones containing the entire human genome is called a 'BAC library.'"

All this comes down to the irrefutable fact that in order to achieve success researchers need to develop effective methods of processing and analyzing massive quantities of information.

Scientists Converged in Massive Effort

In speaking to a 2013 gathering of medical experts, Eric Green, M.D., PhD, director of the National Genome Research Institute, acknowledged that genetics research team members and affiliate organizations need to simplify and streamline the process as much as possible. These should be done despite the massive complexity of the issues involved.

"Our institute recognized this was a huge responsibility; essential to our mission; the date the project ended in 2003, we set the steps to get us down this journey," Green said. "None of us, even the most optimistic people in 2003, envisioned the way that things have progressed the way that they have."

Since then, Green said, researchers have achieved their initial goal of making the effort increasingly sophisticated.

Through each phase of research, and continually as new processes are integrated, the Project has adhered to its five essential objectives:

1. Understanding the structure of genomes
2. Understanding the biology of genomes
3. Understanding the biology of disease
4. Use this to advance the science of medicine
5. Improve the effectiveness of health care

Throughout the process, Green said, participants realized the essential need to continually focus on these core values.

Initial Goals Became Formidable

By 2003, scientists already understood the basic markings or characteristics of the human genome. At that point doctors already knew that the "human blueprint" involves the basic sequencing or ordering of certain universal biological characteristics.

Yet researchers still needed to quantify or decipher the information, specifically to determine what the ordering or sequencing means.

Amazingly, in order to tackle this question, Green said, "one of the tools was to compare it to other genome sequences of other species throughout evolution."

All these became possible thanks to biological research advances from the past several generations. The vast majority of those independent efforts ended by the time that the initial human genome blueprint was finally mapped out. Scientists already knew that people have the same basic building blocks for life contained in all other living earthly species ranging from trees to dogs and chimpanzees.

While any relation between humans and other living creatures might seem ludicrous, the comparisons actually have reaped substantial dividends for genomics science.

Green said that researchers are finally able to catalogue and store the collected data into specific categories. The massive quantities of this information are maintained for future analysis on the Internet, designated for ongoing or subsequent research.

Advancements Occur at Lightning Speed

On the strength of these significant advancements, by 2013 scientists were making milestone genomic and DNA discoveries on a daily basis.

Among their most important findings has been an ongoing determination of which portions of the human genome's sequences are coated in proteins and which are not. This factor, in turn, has accelerated the ability to accurately catalogue data.

Meantime, the continual data analysis has allowed scientists to discover that DNA is actually not so "innocent" or easy to understand as previously believed.

For the first time researchers learned that the DNA of humans is actually a complex "three-dimensional" structure, far more complicated than some scientists previously thought.

A significant discovery came when researchers determined that about one out of every 1,000 of the letters marking the genome sequence is different from the rest. All this, Green said, "has changed the face of genetics research."

To help put this into perspective, before the Human Genome Project began scientists had a clear understanding of just 4,000 of the unique genome signals.

By 2013, researchers had developed systems enabling them to understand the inner workings of 3.4 million markings within the human genome. Scientists continue adding ever-increasing numbers of their findings to the database on a daily basis.

Differences in Humans

The latest research results helped give scientists a much better understanding of why and how each person has a unique overall genetic make-up, when compared to all other individuals.

Scientists believe that herein rests the key to signifying and identifying why and how some people are far more susceptible to specific diseases than others. For instance, some women are genetically predisposed to a greater probability of breast cancer.

By clearly understanding these variations doctors hope to develop cures or preventative procedures for a variety of genetic-related ailments. Besides certain forms of cancer, these range from Alzheimer's Disease and Addison's Disease to Amyotrophic Lateral Sclerosis (ALS), and many more ailments.

Starting from "square one" as if criminal detectives hunting for significant clues, scientists know that each individual person inherits approximately 3 billion genome characteristics from mother and an equal number from the father.

Amazingly, from among the many millions of individual genes already identified, scientists say that they have discovered less than 100 genes that contain "disruptive variants," characteristics that could lead to cures for specific diseases.

5
Significant Cancer Projects Generate Success

Many average consumers worldwide fail to realize that scientists in separate projects across Europe and the United States remain busy making tremendous strides in the battle against cancer--advancements made possible by the Human Genome Project.

With dramatically increased frequency during the next several years cancer patients everywhere are likely to learn of compelling "cures" or remedies made possible by these separate but equally important efforts:

Cancer Genome Project: Thanks to this program, scientists striving to cure cancer worldwide benefit from free online access to critical daily human genomic discoveries. Much of the interest focuses on particularly critical information regarding minute variations in human DNA that lead to the disease. With research facilities based just outside Cambridge, England, the Cancer Genome Project was funded by an independent charity, the London-based Wellcome Trust, now with an endowment of around $20 billion. At the Wellcome Trust Sanger Institute's research facility, this project strives to identify variations and mutations within the human genome sequence that lead to cancer in people. An American-born pharmaceutical magnate, Sir Henry Wellcome founded the trust in 1936, designating the funds for research benefiting animal and human health. These ongoing efforts resulted in scientific technological advancements, accelerating even more upon the fund's 1992 launch of the Sanger Institute. Now the world's second largest charitable fund, behind the Bill and Melinda Gates Foundation, the trust removed all financial interest in the pharmaceutical industry in 1995 by selling its remaining shares in a major drug company. Upon severing its financial ties to the drug industry, the fund began an increasingly important role in "open-source projects," publicly and openly sharing critical information regarding ongoing scientific discoveries, particularly developments relating to the human genome. Starting with its 1992 launch, the Sanger Institute had several primary goals, "a role in mapping, sequencing, and decoding the human genome, and the genomes of other organisms." Scientists say that the Institute made the most significant contribution to what researchers call the "gold standard sequence" of the human genome, before the critical worldwide mapping sequence was completed.

The Cancer Genome Atlas: Funded by the U.S. government, which has close ties to the pharmaceutical industry, the Cancer Genome Atlas is supervised by the National Human Genome Research Institute, and the National Cancer Institute. Starting in 2006, three years after scientists worldwide finished mapping out the human genome, the Cancer Genome Atlas started a three-year pilot project focused on the DNA characteristics of cancers of the ovaries and lungs, plus malignant primary brain tumors in humans called "gioblastoma multiforme." Encouraged by their ability to generate important discoveries from this Phase I research, in 2009 scientists launched a five-year Phase II effort designed to complete a sequence analysis and genomic characterization of up to 25 different tumor types. Wider in scope and more complex than most specialized genomic research projects, Phase II involved at least 500 patient samples--more than most genomics studies, while also using different patient sample analysis techniques. Researchers proclaimed that they had achieved their initial Phase I goal of successfully using various project teams to generate important and statistically valid scientific conclusions. Perhaps just as impressive, the effort's administrators indicated that Phase II had generated a statistically significant data set that will serve as the basis for subsequent essential research.

Hope Reigns Eternal

These formidable efforts generate sincere optimism that doctors someday will control or even "cure" cancer. Yet scientists intricately involved in this vital research admit they lack any specific timeline specifying when such milestones might occur.

Striving to help drive these efforts forward, the National Cancer Institute launched the recently completed Cancer Genome Anatomy Project.

As described by the institute's Website, this effort has "sought to determine the gene expression profiles of normal, pre-cancer and cancer cells, leading eventually to improved detection diagnosis, and treatment for the patient."

In order to achieve success, the institute strives to make this critical information available to the "broad cancer community." Participants include doctors, medical institutions and also researchers continually striving to make significant discoveries.

This highly focused and determined effort enables medical professionals to access essential data on everything from chromosomes, genes, and tissues, to diagrams of biological pathways and protein complexes. Scientists describe these as "links to genetic resources for each known protein."

Along with several other related variables, these vital factors serve as the key attributes regulating how cancer is formed, spreads, grows and eventually tries to kill its "host"--the body of a human being.

Battle Lines Formed

In essence, the entire medical industry serves as a collective army in striving to benefit from human genome discoveries. Call this the "blue" team for hypothetical purposes.

On the opposing side is the proverbial "orange" team, literally the many virulent forms of cancer--particularly the difficult-to-stop varieties that usually kill fast.

Thanks largely to the Cancer Genome Project, the Cancer

Genome Atlas, and the Cancer Genome Anatomy Project, scientists are in the process of doing what all great generals and commanders-in-chief have wanted to do throughout history.

Working together on a consistent, steady basis, researchers are "literally stealing the entire battle plan of this dreaded disease." This informational gathering and processing is steadily enabling doctors to literally know every move or effort made by That Big, Evil Enemy--Cancer.

If this data-collection continues as planned, cancer will literally have little hope of enduring over time. Physicians will know when cancer is more likely to strike specific individuals, particularly people whose genomic profiles indicate such a propensity sometime during life.

Weaponry Created

As more essential data regarding cancer's genomic and DNA characteristics steadily becomes available, researchers also remain busy developing new and more effective treatments. These future remedies have been made possible by recent scientific discoveries.

For these drug-development efforts to work, however, pharmaceutical companies and the researchers advising those firms will need cutting-edge, specific data on minuscule sections of the entire 6-billion strand human genomic sequence.

So, in addition to the various cancer genomic research efforts already mentioned, the U.S. National Institutes of Health (NIH) has created the Cancer Genome Characterization Initiative. According to the Institutes, the Characterization Initiative strives to assess the use of new genomic technologies.

This assessment process serves as a vital way to characterize a subset of genomic changes involved in various types of tumors.

The various agencies, educational institutions and research labs involved in genomic testing all share their data. Participants universally work together with the common goal of successfully describing the many characteristics of cancer.

On a continuous basis the information is recorded in a shared publicly accessible database. The Institute says that while using specific types of genomic analysis, the Initiative employs "second-generation sequencing to better understand the underlying genetic changes leading to cancer."

Important Institution Formed

The Cancer Genome Characterization Initiative database is administered through the NIH's new Office of Cancer Genomics.

Like many of its counterparts in the overall effort cancer genomics research effort, the Office maintains an admirable mission.

As described at the Office's Website, this relatively new institution works to "enhance the understanding of the molecular mechanisms of cancer, advance and accelerate genomics science and technology development, and efficiently translate the genomics data to improve cancer prevention, early detection, diagnosis and treatment."

Besides the separate but related programs already mentioned, the Office administers and monitors several other necessary efforts. Among them:

Cancer Target Discovery and Development: Officials organized this project to bridge what researchers describe as a "gap" between the enormous volumes of genetic data collected and the ability of scientists to develop effective therapeutics. In order to achieve this goal, the project specializes in computational and functional genomics, information essential for sequencing data into usable formats.

TARGET: The designation of "TARGET" is a shortened version of this project's formal name, Therapeutically Applicable Research to Generate Effective Treatments. As described by the TARGET program's Website, this "applies to a comprehensive genomic approach to determine molecular changes that drive childhood cancers." To accomplish this, investigators from numerous agencies and projects form a collaborative effort. They work together to identify and then study specific DNA and genomic characteristics. TARGET is co-managed by divisions of the National Cancer Institute--the previously mentioned Office of Cancer Genomics, and also the Cancer Therapy Evaluation Program.

Major Steps Forward

Taking an aggressive and never-ending approach, these new essential programs operated by the Office of Cancer Genomics follow close on the heels of various initial projects that made the current efforts possible.

In fact, as previously indicated, the Cancer Genome Anatomy Project has already essentially been completed along with several related projects. Each a milestone in humanity's recent formidable discoveries, these now-completed efforts include the:

Initiative for Chemical Genetics: This system used a systematic approach to studying biology through what the Office of Cancer Genomics describes as "small molecule probes and screens, so that new therapies for diseases like cancer can be developed." Like its numerous important counterparts in genomics research, from the onset of its establishment in 2002 this initiative has shared its findings throughout the scientific community. It worked to achieve numerous goals deemed essential in enabling doctors to eventually prevent, treat or eliminate cancer. These tasks included: determining the processes that tumors depend on; determining and identifying the characteristics of "cancer stem cells" that populate tumors; and within the environment of tumors identify the characteristics that promote "metastasis"--the process where cancer spreads to other areas of the body from its initial formation site.

Mammalian Gene Collection: Also operated by the National Institutes of Health, from 2005 to 2009 this project collected, identified and analyzed DNA from a wide variety of mammalian species. Researchers and project administrators said this information was essential to understanding the relationship between humans and other mammals, plus gene characteristics in multiple species that are likely to lead to various physical afflictions or diseases including cancer.

Other Ongoing Efforts

Besides the Cancer Genome Atlas, one of the most significant projects has been the Cancer Genetic Markers of Susceptibility program. Launched in 2005 as a three-year pilot study, this effort sought to identify when, why and how certain individual people inherit a biological susceptibility to acquiring certain types of cancer--such as when the disease initially forms in the breast or other areas.

Sometimes referred to by scientists as "CGEMS," this project developed what the Office of Cancer Genomics describes as a "successful research program." These involved "genome-wide association studies" called "GWAS," striving to identify "genetic variants that affect a person's risk of developing cancer."

Operated by the National Cancer Institute's Division of Cancer Epidemiology and Genetics, the GWAS program relied on information provided by various collaborative epidemiologic studies.

To complete their research, scientists collected bio-specimens of cancers, before scanning the collected DNA for what the program's administrators describe as "cohort or case-control studies."

Thanks to these cutting edge efforts, the scientists were able to identify "inherited genetic variants associated with cancer risk that may lead to new preventative, diagnostic, and therapeutic interventions," the organization says.

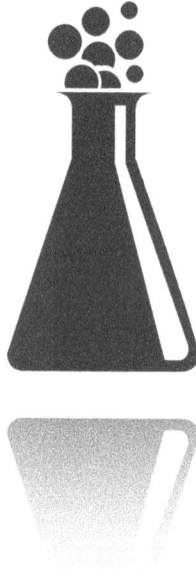

Patients likely will find themselves caught up in the resulting political quagmire, as the "standard medical industry" launches an international propaganda campaign. Consumers everywhere will be told by the "Big Pharma drug industry," that "everything is OK, that cures have been found."

6
Significant Health Care Industry Advancements

Worldwide health care services are on the verge of a significant improvement thanks to genomics research stemming from the "Human Genome Project."

Yet the pharmaceutical industry likely will try to require expensive, dangerous, harmful and often addictive drugs as a result of this huge international effort.

Conversely, fighting for the good health and rights of patients everywhere, Homeopaths who practice natural medicine will enter the fray with harmless, inexpensive natural remedies.

Patients likely will find themselves caught up in the resulting political quagmire, as the "standard medical industry" launches an international propaganda campaign. Consumers everywhere will be told by the "Big Pharma drug industry," that "everything is OK, that cures have been found."

Sadly, however, I fear that in all likelihood many drugs identified by genomics research as "cures for specific diseases" actually will generate harmful side effects. This likely would happen, particularly if the miserable past performance of the multi-billion-dollar drug industry is any indication of future results.

You see, as previously indicated, the standard medical profession in the United States is closely tied to Big Pharma, which has cronies inside all health-related federal agencies. Worsening matters on a massive scale, some of these same agencies are intricately involved in critical ongoing genomics research.

Shockingly, this little-known behind-the-scenes battle has never been reported in-depth by the mainstream news media. The big "loser" here has been the general public, which has lacked any inkling that their health--and literally their lives--could hinge in the balance of back-room political skulduggery.

Brave New World

Future advancements might emerge as reminiscent of Aldous Huxley's classic 1931 novel, "Brave New World," unless the influence of Big Pharma on genomic research is counter-balanced with natural remedies. Huxley's book, often heralded as among the 100 best novels of the 20th Century, anticipates future significant technology developments that negatively impact society.

Comparing the current dilemma with the potential dangers specified in Huxley's classic is no stretch of the imagination. This predicament continues worsening, particularly when taking into account the fact that Big Pharma within the USA has shown a consistent reckless disregard for the public.

Most of the many domestic-based genomic research projects work in conjunction with federal agencies.

With this critical feature clearly understood, it would be ludicrous to think that key decision makers who lead genomics research would ultimately specify as treatments the many natural, harmless and effective remedies found worldwide in Mother Nature.

As previously stated, I'm among Homeopaths who fear that instead of identifying and recommending natural remedies, these officials likely will hinge their research and ultimately their recommendations primarily on manmade synthetic drugs.

Ultimately, I worry that all this would come at a horrific cost, perhaps generating incalculable levels of suffering throughout the middle class and poor worldwide.

Discover a Terrifying New World

Imagine an international economy where only the rich and super-wealthy are guaranteed so-called "cures" from the most deadly and crippling diseases.

Within this new realm that some people might justifiably label the "Terrifying New World," pharmaceutical companies charge exorbitant rates for the only synthetic drugs deemed effective for a specific disease such as cancer of the pancreas.

At present, according to an article in "American Family Physician," the current survival rate for people suffering from cancer of the pancreas is only 2 percent to 9 percent.

Yet envision a future "Terrifying New World," where findings generated by genomics research result in a new unnatural synthetic drug that generates a pancreatic tumor survival rate of nearly 100 percent.

Right away this might seem like fantastic news, particularly for people suffering from the disease and for their loved ones.

Disturbingly, what if Big Pharma implements over-the-moon fees of tens of thousands of dollars per patient for the "one-and-only, government certified Official Cures" of such catastrophic or fatal conditions?

Ailing consumers and their families would suffer from extreme cases of "Sticker Shock."

Forget the Law of "Supply and Demand"

Following their usual practice of overcharging the way they already do today, Big Pharma very likely would impose fees far surpassing the ability of most consumers and large insurance companies to pay.

Under worst-case scenarios, the cost of a single round of "cure drugs" for the most deadly diseases would exceed the combined amounts that a single consumer could earn over several years.

Essentially, advance-stage cancer patients everywhere would be told, "Pay Up, or Die." In essence without necessarily saying so in such specific words, Big Pharma would essentially "own your ability to survive, unless you're willing and able to pay."

Without exaggeration, particularly among those of us highly familiar with the selfish strategies of Big Pharma, to forecast per-patient fees of $150,000 for so-called "cure drugs" would be far from science fiction--but rather an "everyday reality."

As haunting as this might sound, only the rich or politically connected would have any good chance of survival from Stage IV cancer when visiting a mainstream physician. This would hold true even within the era of Obamacare, a dismal failure at improving the U.S. health insurance system while also ravaging the entire medical industry.

Healthy People Suffer

Adding fuel to the proverbial fire, many people currently enjoying good, vibrant health also would suffer financially--in some cases to a horrific degree.

These instances will stem from the fact genomics research efforts are identifying and locating specific types of harmful genes in healthy infants, children and young adults.

Certain genetic markers indicate that they are likely to contract future ailments ranging from breast cancer to Alzheimer's Disease. Perhaps dozens or hundreds of potential future health issues will be identified.

As a result, once again would Big Pharma benefit unless natural and harmless remedies are found and developed?

From the perspective of many consumers, "Big Brother will own me--my actual body. The government, the medical industry and especially Big Pharma will behave as if I am their physical property--all while under the bogus, deceptive guise of having my well being and my personal welfare as their highest priority."

Big Pharma's Reckless Record

The overall pharmaceutical industry has earned a well-deserved reputation for ineptitude. Along with greed, selfishness and recklessness, some of the many "sins" of Big Pharma already include:

Side effects: Knowingly and willfully manufacturing and

66

distributing drugs with extremely harmful side effects, selling to consumers who never realize the full potential negative impacts of such danger.

Addiction: Propagating or accepting a distribution and sales system that enables doctors to recklessly prescribe medications or painkillers that lead to drug dependency.

Costs: Particularly within the United States, forces consumers to pay ridiculously high per-pill fees--sometimes up to $8,000 per dose, and in many instances much more.

Politics: Contributes tens of millions of dollars in campaign funds to the USA's congressional and presidential candidates, thereby obliterating any and all potentially effective political dissent.

Lobbyists: Big Pharma employs tens of thousands of high-power lobbyists, most in Washington, D.C., the USA's epicenter of political decisions.

Cronies: The nation's medical school staffs, hospitals, general mainstream doctors and health-related federal agency bureaucracies are loaded with medical professionals who have been brainwashed. While dissent among these ranks is rare, as an overall group these individuals are trained to blindly put all their faith and hope in Big Pharma.

Fully cognizant of these many destructive factors, why would consumers believe that "everything will be OK?" Why would the general population say, "We should put all of our faith and trust in them? Surely they have our welfare in mind?"

Medical Center

Name

Address

Date

R
X

Shockingly, some apparent Big Pharma cronies have even gone so far as to propose that doctors be required to quantify and input the DNA and genomic make-up of every newborn in the United States within 48 hours of birth.

MD

Signature

7
Social Nightmares

As if the many issues already mentioned were already
ample reason to suffer nightmares, an additional factor emerges--
scary enough to send shivers down the spine.

Once again reminiscent of Huxley's "Brave New World,"
in conformance with federal law mandated by Obamacare,
every time an individual's DNA or entire genome is measured
that person's data will have to be placed in a universal national
database.

Shockingly, some apparent Big Pharma cronies have even
gone so far as to propose that doctors be required to quantify and
input the DNA and genomic make-up of every newborn in the
United States within 48 hours of birth.

Doctors and insurance companies, plus perhaps even the
IRS, would have access to the sensitive personal data. At face
value, all this might sound harmless and to the great benefit of
medical researchers striving to compile accurate data.

Yet nothing could be further from the case.

Labeled as "Damaged Goods"
Yes, imagine the anguish suffered by a child or young adult
"marked as broken" while the person remains healthy--all because
DNA markers indicate the individual has a biological propensity
for suffering heart disease or other serious ailment starting later in
life.

A huge unwanted potential would become being branded
as an "unusable, worthless biological mass."

You see, every doctor that the person visits throughout
life will have full access to the database. The fact that hackers
likely will try to steal the information exacerbates this horrendous
problem multi-fold.

Everyday people, and particularly celebrities, could very well find themselves as hopeless victims of the criminal underworld.

Besides the threat of potential blackmail, what if hackers end up selling your personal genomic information on the black market?

Once again, these real-life issues could spiral out of control in a society where such a scenario once had been considered "mere science fiction."

Withholding Crucial Information

On the positive side, at this point there seems to be no solid evidence that any official will intentionally withhold a "negative DNA diagnosis" from any person.

To do so surely should be classified as a serious criminal offense, perhaps even a felony, particularly in instances where such information indicates a future fatal disease.

Yet why would anyone or any institution withhold such information?

Well, the answer is actually quite simple--while also highly disturbing.

Within the so-called "Wicked New World," what if institutions or groups of individuals emerge in the medical industry who consider themselves as the ultimate Death Panel?

Under such a worst-case scenario, such an organization would bestow upon itself the crucial decision of "determining who should live, and who should die."

While such a suggestion might seem preposterous today, modern consumers need to realize that the United States government has a verified history of making reckless, cruel and demonic life-and-death decisions.

As ludicrous as this might sound, it's true. At the Nevada Nuclear Test site during the 1950s and 1960s the federal government ignited above-ground nuclear bombs, all while telling the gullible public that "everything is perfectly safe--there is nothing to worry about."

Yet government documents uncovered in the late 20th Century revealed that federal agencies actually knew all along that the nuclear fallout was extremely deadly to the civilian population unlucky enough to be downwind of the blasts.

Tens of thousands of people within the fallout zone suffered from cancer in the decades that followed, far surpassing the normal rate for the disease within society. By an act of Congress, in the 1990s many families that had lived in the nuclear fallout zones several decades earlier received financial compensation from the federal government. These payments were designated as "a payback for their pain and suffering." But the physical, emotional and economic damage had already been done.

So, why now should we be expected to the put our full faith and trust in the U.S. government in regard to the storage and distribution of DNA test results?

Destructive Propaganda

Aided by the naive and often lazy mainstream news media, allopathic physicians who prescribe dangerous, expensive and addictive Big Pharma drugs continually portray Homeopaths that administer natural remedies "as quacks involved in a useless profession."

While continuing to disseminate this irresponsible propaganda, the bulk of mainstream physicians in the United States apparently would like to prohibit Homeopaths from developing effective, natural treatments stemming from genomics research.

If that happened, the so-called Big Winners would become the greedy, selfish and reckless giant pharmaceutical companies. On the losing end, consumers across the United States and perhaps worldwide would be "stuck with" what standard doctors tell them is the only effective option for treatment--Big Pharma drugs.

Such an outcome is highly predictable, particularly when accounting for the previous and ongoing propaganda

71

efforts launched by the mainstream medical industry in soiling the reputation of medical professionals who administer natural remedies.

Primary Issue Emerges

Herein rests the primary issue, namely that purely for financial gain, natural substances would never be considered as effective treatments for specific ailments identified by genomics research.

Such a scenario emerges from the fact that Big Pharma is unable to apply for and receive patents on harmless and effective natural substances found naturally in great abundance. Such remedies would fail to generate huge profits.

When working in conjunction with federal agencies like the FDA, is there a likelihood that mainstream doctors would block any effort by genomics research to identify effective natural substances?

Do you think mainstream doctors would have the general public's welfare in mind, or would these physicians favor their allies closely tied to Big Pharma?

A huge danger exists, namely that behind-the-scenes insider politics could very well play a key role in identifying genomics-related remedies--without the general public ever realizing that drug company allies are "literally playing with their lives."

8
Mastering Human Traits

In order for genomics research to conquer extremely rare diseases such as Cystic Fibrosis, the so-called "trick" rests in determining how these unusual variants determine an individual's unique traits--also known as "phenotypes." Although genetically simple on a biological level, until now the underlying characteristics have been extremely difficult to identify because they involve defects in a single gene.

The discovery rate has been far greater in identifying monogenic diseases or traits, characteristics that lead to ailments found much more commonly in general populations. As of 2013, scientists had identified about 5,000 disease-related genes.

Through that year the proverbial glass was "half full," as more than 1,600 successful genome-wide studies continued to advance what scientists know about the impact of the human DNA make-up on disease.

Much of the current focus centers on portions of the human genome that are not coated in proteins, a process described by some experts as challenging and intimidating.

Target Specific Patients

Rather than determine how specific genome sequences operate, researchers and doctors want to know how such biological processes work within individual patients. This way experts hope to eventually address each person's specific health issues.

Once again, according to the top administrators of the biggest, most significant genomics research projects, the key here likely rests in determining and quantifying the full range of sequences that lack protein coating. Getting a full understanding here can only occur when scientists complete genome inventories of individual people in specific groups, each containing members who suffer from a specific ailment.

As this whole-genome sequencing aspect of the entire effort began in April 2003, scientists reported that they needed "technical leaps that seemed so far off as to almost be fictional, but which--if they could be achieved--would revolutionize biomedical research and clinical practice."

A related initial goal also was to significantly reduce the cost of determining the entire DNA sequence within a single individual. As genomics research entered its current phase during 2003, computer models suggested this expense would be around $6.5 million per person--significantly above the researchers' long-term goal of just $1,000.

Amazingly, according to research administrators by 2013 the cost had dipped to around $8,000 per individual thanks to widespread technological advances, some that stemmed from results obtained through trial and error after the scientists completed the genome map.

Remember that by now, as previously stated officials say the ongoing research is well on its way to achieving its goal of lowering the cost to $1,000 for each patient. This, in turn, could very well emerge as a significant advancement, vastly increasing the potential numbers of people who can benefit from advances in genomics medicine at the point that the research identifies effective treatments.

New Doctors Need Vital Info
As effective genomics-generated treatments emerge, leaders of the medical industry admit they're faced with the additional challenge of easily incorporating the findings into the educational system.

With steadily increasing importance, the overriding task remains determining how to train the next generation of physicians to analyze and use the data that they find.

As envisioned by today's researchers, some day doctors will be able to order an affordable entire genome scan of an individual patient--before determining which specific drugs or treatments, if any, are required for that patient.

The hope here among genomic researchers is that someday doctors, perhaps as early as the 2030s or 2040s, will have a tried-and-true protocol to follow. If all "goes well," by that point getting a complete genome scan for a person will become as prevalent and commonly used as standard, typical blood tests are today.

Within a day or so of getting their personal genomes mapped out, patients could be informed about the apparent underlying cause of their specific ailment. Under typical scenarios, doctors would then strive to follow criteria or protocol as officially mandated by the medical industry.

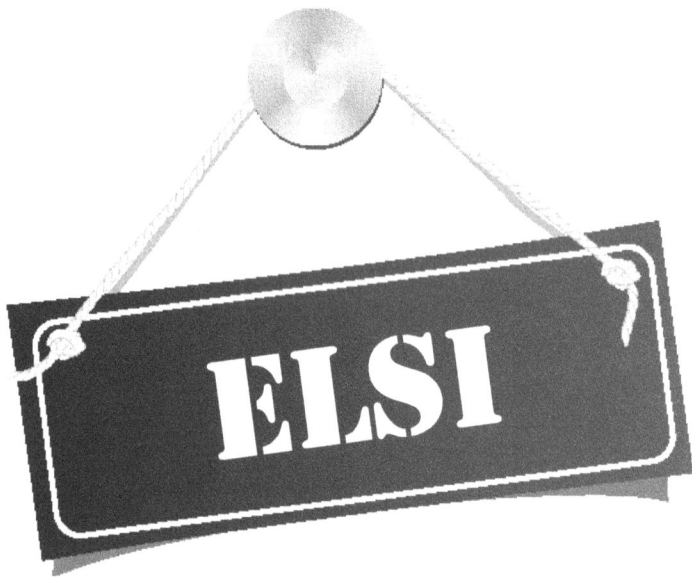

Claiming to strive for "high moral ground" on ethical issues, administrators of the genomics research allied to Big Pharma have created an infrastructure designed to address any "ethical, legal and social issues" that might arise. Bureaucrats have labeled this ELSI.

9
More Potential Dangers and Benefits: New Drugs Will Emerge

Although many analysts might predict otherwise, consumers can expect numerous all-new drugs to emerge as a result of genomics research stemming from the Project.

On an official basis, at least according to its Website genome.gov, new drugs developed as a result of the studies will emerge around 2020 to 2025.

The Food and Drug Administration reported that by 2010 at least 350 new biotech products were undergoing clinical trials. Staffed largely by Big Pharma allies, the FDA usually takes at least a decade to give a new drug final approval, beginning when research starts.

Under ideal situations, the best and most effective drugs that win approval during these initial phases would be used as a "preventative measure" for people whose genome scans indicate that they face the danger of specific future ailments.

This, in turn, could emerge as a huge and almost unstoppable boom for drug companies. Imagine the tremendous profits generated for Big Pharma when patients are button-holed into using the only options given--pharmaceutical products.

Ethical Issues Muddy the Waters

Claiming to strive for "high moral ground" on ethical issues, administrators of the genomics research allied to Big Pharma have created an infrastructure designed to address any "ethical, legal and social issues" that might arise. Bureaucrats have labeled this ELSI.

For many decades the ELSI system is supposed to monitor potential issues, deciding how doctors, pharmacies, drug makers and genomics researchers should respond to specific types of situations.

Ultimately the panel or documentation is supposed to determine what is "right and wrong," concerning pivotal and potential controversial matters ranging from patient rights to what drugs are deemed proper for protocols that doctors will have to follow.

Yet from the perspective of consumer rights, could this "Ethics-Cop System" be like "putting the foxes in charge of the henhouse?" Can Big Pharma allies be trusted to place the patients' health and personal finances higher on priority lists than pharmaceutical company profits?

Keep in mind that any specific events or processes that one person thinks is "just and fair," could simultaneously be viewed by another individual as "unjust and unfair."

The supposed morality of ethics remains a cloudy undertaking, and those running the system of dictating "morals and the right way to do things" are likely to rule in their own favor. The danger here is that power-hungry Big Brother essentially will operate in his own favor.

Beware of Big Pharma's Power

Project administrators consider current and future ethical issues as so important that they have set aside 5 percent of the system's budget to handle ethical, legal and social issues. The panel or its bureaucrats are in charge of providing guidance for "policymakers" and the public.

Well, if the past is any indication of future performance, those who run genomics research--complying with the dictates of Big Pharma--would essentially issue strong recommendations to Congress on what laws to pass. New regulations would protect the drug makers' financial interests, while essentially ignoring concerns vital to consumers. In all likelihood government would relieve the companies of potential liability.

If and when that happens everyday consumers would essentially find themselves with little or no options regarding their personal health care.

At least as viewed from the eyes of some observers, all this might look like the type of fictional horror story reminiscent of "zombie movies" where all living humans might fight continually to protect themselves. Yet the major corporations allied to politicians and mainstream medicine would actually be "running the show," a blood-curdling horror story.

Top all this off with a system that refuses to consider consumer complaints, and people everywhere within the United States would truly become helpless, dependent and victimized wards of the state. Truly your life would be "in their hands."

Morality Issues Run Amok

Essentially by putting all the so-called moral power within the hands of the government and genomics research administrators, streams of vital issues could very well come to play, with the public given little or no say in policy. Among just some of the many issues:

Costs: With Big Pharma essentially helping to "run the show," expect little or no checks and balances regulating or prohibiting super-high drug costs.

Live or Die: Essentially washing their hands of any potential liability, mainstream doctors and Big Pharma could proclaim that they're simply following policy in determining who should be allowed to live and who should die.

Adverse side effects: Just as they do now with protocol that requires the use of poisonous chemo for advanced Stage IV cancer patients, when genetics research generates new drugs allopathic doctors will state that they are "just following the rules"--thereby getting automatic relief from potential liability stemming from known adverse side effects.

Personal privacy: Consumers supposedly would be given a guarantee that their personal information stemming from genome tests shall remain hidden. But just as federal bureaucrats have done with Obamacare, such sensitive information would be left vulnerable to theft on the Internet--open to hackers.

Pre-Employment Tests: A primary fear stems from the fact that potential employers might refuse to hire anyone whose personal genome scan indicates that his or her DNA indicates a propensity for future disease. Employers might say otherwise, but doctors who represent those companies would have access to extremely sensitive personal information.

10
Government Controls Your Health

Following a pattern first installed by Obamacare, the U.S. government would essentially be taking charge of everyone's personal health issues via genomic research.

Of course, some liberal politicians strive to proclaim otherwise, deceptively making the bogus claim that the law regulates health insurance--rather than health care.

Hopefully such smoke-and-mirrors tactics would fail to fool most of today's savvy consumers, when and if politicians and bureaucrats twist genomics-related rules in favor of Big Pharma. Yet with bureaucrats calling the shots, little could be done to stem the dangerous tide from swamping consumers.

You see, within today's corrupt American political system, only Big Money talks in a way guaranteed to make politicians "listen and take sides." Herein rests the vital key to success for cash-laden, multi-billion-dollar pharmaceutical companies-- campaign donations.

Yet sadly only super-wealthy individuals and mega-corporations like those ensconced within Big Pharma can afford sizable political campaign contributions.

Once again, as previously indicated, the situation might seem somewhat hopeless or even a lost cause when adding to this the disturbing fact that most of today's consumers lack any inkling of what is truly going on behind the scenes.

Who could blame everyday citizens for their apparent ignorance on these issues? After all, as exemplified by the many examples already listed, just like Obamacare did while in its own initial implementation phase, the ethical issues ensconced within genomics research are numerous, complex and intermixed.

Only a handful of Americans are likely to delve deeply into such issues, let alone try to take decisive action to fight any existing or potential provisions. Worsening matters, even if they launch a cohesive opposition to Big Pharma strategies, everyday consumers would lack the necessary financial resources to make their quest effective.

Initial Propaganda Emerges

Launching an early strike in the clandestine propaganda war, the National Human Genome Research Institute states unequivocally that it is ethical, legal and socially necessary. The Institute says this effort "provides an effective basis from which to assess the implications of genome research, and has resulted in several notable improvements."

Claiming that its ELSI program serves as a model for large, publicly funded science efforts, the Institute likely will have many more questions to answer if the mainstream general public ever catches wind of what is happening behind closed doors.

"Molecularizing disease and their possible impact will have a profound impact on what patients expect from medical help and the new generation of doctors' perception of illness," said a 2000 article by H.J. Rheinberger in the Cambridge University Press.

Meantime, however, there seems to be no significant, vocal and widespread opposition to the biggest genomics research projects, at least on moral grounds.

The gullible and often ill-informed general public seems to convey a message via its relentless silence: "We do not care enough to get involved. Do with us what you will, dear government."

Many Health Issues Addressed

To their great credit, overall the individuals involved in the Project seem to be showing a supreme and tremendous dedication to improving health care.

Indeed, the many scientists, doctors and researchers deserve great praise for their individual and combined efforts.

Keep in mind that the overall stated and primary goal of the genomics research is to develop knowledge and treatments designed to improve and maintain good health. Such efforts are certainly worthy of praise on a worldwide scale.

"Overall, the underlying goal of genomics research is nothing short of tremendous," I tell any patient who might ask for my opinion on the issue.

"Excluding the many real or potential problems involving drugs, the many research efforts' underlying goals are nothing short of revolutionary."

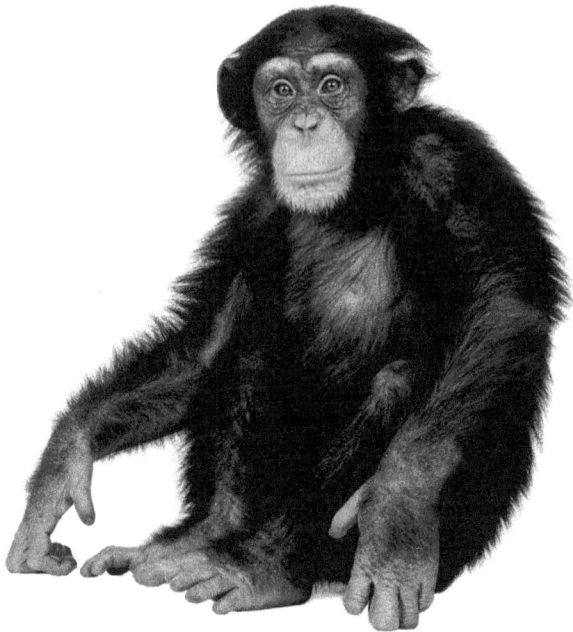

Humans vs. Apes

The genome mapping process has enabled
scientists to determine that a mere nine genetic
differences separate humans from chimpanzees.

11
Chimpanzee Genome Project

A key and important segment of the overall effort to advance genomic medicine involved the Chimpanzee Genome Project. Researchers mapped the entire genome sequence of the chimp primate, before methodically comparing those results to the structure within humans.

Scientists say that people are different than other primates in a genetic sense because humans have 23 chromosomes. By comparison, apes including chimpanzees have 24 chromosomes.

This intense research phase hinges largely on the fact that most scientists believe in evolution, the controversial theory first proposed by Charles Darwin in the 19th Century. Darwin theorized that certain apes evolved into modern humans.

That's in sharp contrast with the basic religious belief systems including Christianity, which maintains that God made the first man--Adam--out of clay.

The philosophical and heated controversy took an interesting twist in October 2014, when Pope Francis--international leader of the Roman Catholic Church--mystified and upset many conservative Christians by proclaiming that evolution occurred.

Aside from such philosophical and spiritual discussion, scientists do their job by concentrating on facts as they view them within the perceived or measurable universe. To them, the evolutionary evidence from genetic material collected from multiple eras over hundreds of millions of years appear to demonstrate that modern humans gradually evolved from other primates--although the religious controversy continues.

Basic Evolution Evolved

From the basic overall view of the mainstream scientific

community, most mammalian species steadily evolve over extended time in order to adapt to each specific animal's survival requirements.

For instance, scientists say that in the cold and snowy antarctic, white polar bears steadily evolved into their present appearance. Having brown or black fur would have made polar bears too easy for their intended prey to spot in snowy or icy environments. A white appearance makes polar bears more successful than brown or black bears would be within the arctic wild.

In a similar overall evolutionary pattern, yet for much different reasons, modern humans gradually obtained larger brains. The brains of people are significantly bigger percentage-wise in relation to overall body mass, when compared to most other mammals.

Scientists say that several hundred million years ago such changes in brain size and body structure of certain early apes was barely noticeable from one generation to the next. Yet over time, a subset of those primates needed to obtain a greater intelligence in order to survive, endure and thrive within rapidly changing environments.

Scientists say that thanks largely to these epic changes, as a species humans were able to survive through numerous catastrophic global events. The most recent was the last Ice Age, which ended about 10,000 years ago.

Humans vs. Apes

The genome mapping process has enabled scientists to determine that a mere nine genetic differences separate humans from chimpanzees.

This emerges as far from a joking matter to researchers. They insist that clearly understanding this aspect of the evolutionary process could lead to a far greater knowledge of the human genome--ultimately enabling scientists to discover how to optimize health for all people.

The hope remains that by intricately detailing how ape-to-human evolution occurred, scientists will obtain a far better understanding of how the entire genome of a person should look for optimal health.

Eager to make these vital comparisons, researchers immediately created the Chimpanzee Genome Project as scientists finished mapping the entire human genome. The chimp effort's initial researchers worked at a break-neck pace. They completed the initial mapping of the entire chimpanzee genome sequence in December 2003, a mere eight months after announcing that the entire human genome blueprint had been "mapped out."

Only in a modern sense, think of this as an old-style dot-to-dot game in which children simply "connect the dots." At the start everything looks like a mere hodgepodge, random and unrelated marks on a page or screen.

Chimpanzee Work Intensified

With each new month since late 2003, scientists have gained a far greater understanding of the unique genetic differences between humans and apes.

By 2013 researchers began using data amassed through the Chimpanzee Genome Project to estimate that the evolution from ape to modern human took 7 million years--a mere "speck" of time in a universal sense.

Also, while all current life in many forms and species is distantly related to each other, the genetic make-up of humans is far more similar to chimps than to any other animal.

Despite these minuscule differences, some of the the most significant changes in the biology of humans transpired in the past 250,000 years. That is considered a relatively brief period in relation to the age of the earth, by some accounts 4.5 billion years old.

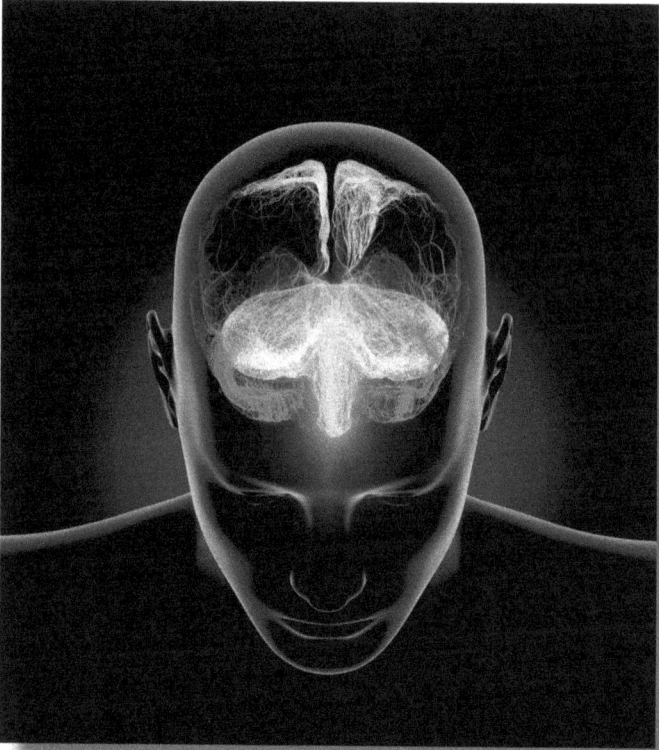

Doctors hope the Brain Project will determine the specific roots of a vast array of destructive and sometimes deadly diseases that start within that essential organ.

12

Various Side Projects Emerged

Numerous other side projects commenced, beginning shortly after the 2003 completion of the human genome map.

Scientists became increasingly determined to launch and continue vital and significant research. These programs are likely to individually and collectively result in discoveries and cures for specific types of afflictions or diseases that attack certain bodily areas. Among some of the most important programs:

Human Brain Project

The Human Brain Project was finalized in 2013, a full decade after the primary Human Genome Project's mapping phase ended.

Primarily funded by The European Union, the Human Brain Project is using supercomputers in an effort to mimic that organ's vital functions within humans.

By accomplishing this formidable feat, scientists believe that they'll gain a far greater understanding of the integral functioning within the human brain.

Based in Switzerland, this subset of the overall project has many important long-term goals, such as specifically understanding how the brain reacts to certain drugs.

Of just as much or perhaps even greater importance, doctors hope the Brain Project will determine the specific roots of a vast array of destructive and sometimes deadly diseases that start within that essential organ.

Hopefully, important clues uncovered during the next few decades will enable researchers to develop methods for: healing brain injury; understanding how the brain evolves and matures during the phases of life; and developing effective treatments for specific ailments ranging from dementia to Parkinson's Disease.

Also, as unbelievable as this might seem, it's true--

the Human Brain Project's other notable goals include the development of high-end computer chips.

Expect Significant Advancements

If the Brain Project makes discoveries that scientists hope for, the effort will generate world-changing technological advancements destined to change the future course of human civilization. Among the most significant:

Energy savings: Develop super-fast computers that minimize the need for energy with each minuscule calculation that results in the transfer of data.

Neuroscience: Develop a complete understanding of every aspect of the human nervous system that regulates all functions within the body.

Interdisciplinary effort: Develop a keen understanding of mathematics, linguistics, genetics, engineering, chemistry, medicine and computer science.

Allied disciplines: Other targets for research and development include psychology, physics and philosophy.

Broadened approach: Sometimes used interchangeably with the term "neurobiology," the overall field of neuroscience also has grown to include approaches to computational, evolutionary, developmental, structural and mental functions.

Neuromorphic Computing: First developed in the late 1980s, this scientific discipline involves the large-scale integration of analog circuits that mimic neurobiological structures. This could result in significant advancements in robots, ultimately enabling such devices to move as if human, perhaps calculating, storing and deciphering data in much the same way as people.

Robotic Advancements

According to a wide variety of published reports, numerous significant advancements in robotry have resulted from genetic research.

First, results derived from the Human Genome Project

gave scientists an understanding of how computations are derived from the human genome's overall: design; biological circuits; and the interactions and functions of neurons. These potential robotics advancements involve a branch of biology called "morphology," the study of the specific structural features and forms of organisms.

A vast array of scientific research branches each have specific and individualized studies of morphology. These include linguistics, astronomy, archaeology and many other scientific disciplines.

Within biology, scientists have numerous specific fields of study, most or all of them significantly improved thanks to the Human Genome Project and the Human Brain Project. These include:

Experimental Morphology: Using experimental conditions to determine the effect of "external factors" such as the impacts of genetic mutations.

Functional Morphology: The study of the function and structure of the overall "morphology of an organism," how the various cells interact.

Comparative Morphology: Analyzing all structures within the individual, ultimately defining and naming specific groups of biological organisms.

Criticisms Emerged

Although the Human Brain Project's overall goals seem admirable, some scientists have questioned the ability of this segment of the overall effort to meet its goals.

In a document sent to the European Commission on July 7, 2014, at least 595 researchers signed an advisory notifying officials that the Brain Project has an "overly narrow" approach-generating a significant risk that the effort will fail to meet its goals.

Complaints stemmed from a decision by an administrator at the Swiss Federal Institute of Technology, Henry Markram.

Some cognitive scientists claim policies implemented by Markram sidelined researchers who specialize in high-level brain functions like thought and behavior; they threatened to boycott the Brain Project due to Markram's controversial administrative changes.

Reporting in a July 2014 article about the threatened boycott, "The Guardian" said that Peter Dayan, director of computational neuroscience at University College in London, believes that any large-scale simulation of the brain would be radically premature.

Even so, another report to the European Commission indicated that the Brain Project likely will result in lower-cost advanced medical options for patients.

Also, as previously stated, perhaps just as impressive-- at least from the apparent viewpoint of consumers--the Human Brain Project ultimately could result in earlier and better treatment methods and diagnostic technology.

Meantime, however, reports to the European Commission also list numerous "obstacles" or challenges facing the Brain Project. Potential hurdles here stem from the methodology in collecting and storing data from previous biological and DNA research.

Varying institutions used different research efforts, development stages, species and methodology. This, in turn, has resulted in the difficult task of quantifying the overall information.

More Ethical Dilemmas Emerged

Like the overall U.S.-based Human Genome Project, the Europe-based Human Brain Project has generated questions regarding the touchy issue of "ethics."

Once again, society is faced with a potential clash of cultures and belief systems, where some groups believe that conducting genomics brain research is flat-out morally "right"-- while others insist that such efforts are "wrong" and unethical.

The Brain Project's administration says that the effort maintains a "Responsible Innovation" policy. Herein emerge significant considerations, namely vital questions of what should and will be deemed as either "responsible" or "irresponsible." For the Brain Project, such efforts are overseen by the "Ethics and Society Programme," which has various committees.

Key among these are the Ethical, Legal and Social Aspects Committee, plus the Research Ethics Committee--responsible for determining how data is collected, the treatment of animals used in research, and the collection of data from people.

The Blue Brain Project

Formally unaffiliated with the Human Brain Project, the "Blue Brain Project," uses a Switzerland facility and research project in an attempt to use reverse-engineering to create a human brain that functions precisely at the molecular level.

Designed to study the brain's functional and architectural principles, the Blue Brain Project was formed in May 2005 by part of the Swiss Federal Institute of Technology, École polytechnique fédérale de Lausann.

Founded by the Swiss federal government, the school serves as a hub for interaction between industry and the scientific community. Besides educating scientists and engineers, the institution strives to serve as a national center for excellence in science and technology.

Reminiscent of the disturbing plot of "Brave New World," the Blue Brain Project involves a blue-green supercomputer. The technology uses what scientists call "neuron software" that simulates environments for modeling networks of neurons and individual neurons.

In biology, neurons serve an essential role in the vital process of electrically excitable cells, enabling them to transmit and process vital information. Using chemical and electrical signals, neurons use "synapse," a process enabling the transfer of chemical or electrical signals to other cells.

Using data input by researchers, the supercomputer or "blue brain" strives to mimic the functioning and neuron communication process of humans. This involves the reverse-engineering process that strives to extract information about design or knowledge from anything that is manmade.

Scientists analyze the components and functions of individual biological units. They also use reverse-engineering to determine how certain biological invaders are structured. The resulting data enables researchers to devise methods of removing or blocking electrical signals.

Strive for "Realism"

The Blue Brain Project strives to use a "biologically realistic" model of neurons, in order to mimic human brain function as much as possible.

Scientists are so optimistic that some researchers hope the effort will eventually reveal details about the nature of consciousness, according to a 2012 article in "The Hebrew University of Jerusalem."

The overall Blue Brain Project is so diverse and increasingly widespread that the effort has spawned numerous sub-projects at various other educational institutions worldwide.

These include the Supercomputing and Visualization Center of Madrid's Cajal Blue Brain, all coordinated by the Technical University of Madrid. This sub-project has its own unique sets of computer simulations and neurological experimentations.

In December 2006, separate from but related to the overall Human Brain Project, the Blue Brain Project simulated the neocortical column within rats. Some scientists consider the column as the smallest biological component of the neocortex, the largest part of the cerebral cortex within mammalian brains.

Intricate Biological Beauty

To understand the importance of the Blue Brain Project,

keep in mind that humans use the neocortex for higher brain functions such as:

Sensory perception: The vital and essential uses of sight, hearing, taste, smell, and touch--plus the ability to sense temperature, pain and balancing needs.

Motor commands: This gives a person the ability to voluntarily and intentionally move body parts--planning, controlling and executing each action.

Spatial reasoning: Sometimes called "spatial visualization ability," this gives a healthy person the ability to sense the distance, placement and size of objects.

Conscious thought: Commonly called "consciousness," this entails the process of being "aware" or knowing about oneself or an external object. While having a "sense of self," the individual has a sense of awareness or subjectivity.

Obtaining intricate knowledge on the structure, functions and inter-workings of these functions would truly emerge as a remarkable achievement.

Such research could truly generate groundbreaking discoveries, especially when realizing that a single functional unit of the neocortex within humans has a whopping 60,000 neurons. Each neocortex unit has a diameter of only 0.5 millimeters.

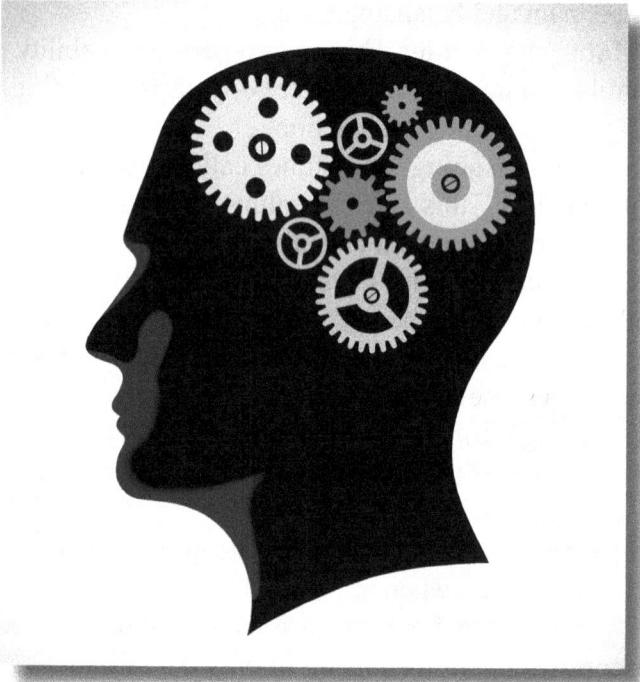

Scientists say that artificial neural networks have already been used to perform tasks such as speech recognition, and also generating the ability of "sight" in which machines understand, analyze and process images.

13
The Mind-Boggling Decade of the 2020s

According to documentation released by Markram, by 2023 scientists should be able to model the entire structure of the estimated 100 billion cells in the human brain.

When and if researchers achieve this goal, they should be able to construct a simulation of the entire human brain on a molecular level, according to a June 2005 article in "New Scientist."

Researchers yearn to use such a model for their ongoing studies, largely because such a tool would enable them to identify the effects of a process that scientists call "gene expression." This occurs as a result of "synthesis," when two or more entities or objects combine to form something new.

Gene expression results in the formation of a functional gene product, either a protein or RNA. These microscopic units are essential to the formation and the specific characteristics of life.

Formed by one or more long chains of amino acid residues, proteins serve a vast array of functions within organisms. Primary activities include responding to stimuli and replicating DNA in order to create healthy new cells when "old cells" naturally die on a continual basis.

For scientists involved in the Blue Brain Project, another critical goal involves the simulation of multiple connected neocortical columns. Such an achievement ultimately would enable them to simulate the function of an entire neocortex.

Lightning-Fast Advancements

Various significant and intermingled sub-projects have emerged partly as a result of the Blue Brain Project. Among them:

Artificial Brain: This involves the development of

hardware and software that possesses and uses human-like cognitive abilities. As previously mentioned, this would give researchers a better understanding of cognitive science. The creation of such a structure could eventually generate two world-changing technological developments. The first of these is the ability to experiment with "the philosophy of artificial intelligence;" such a process would give researchers the ability to demonstrate if a scientific theory accurately forecasts that humans have the ability to create machines having the abilities of people. The second significant development would involve determining the possibility of creating machines that replicate animals including humans, particularly the complex nervous system. Already progressing at a fairly brisk pace, scientists at such institutions as Aston University in Birmingham, England, have already used various processes to create biological cells called "neurospheres." Comprised of small clusters of neurons, these structures are used in laboratory settings to determine their effectiveness in addressing such afflictions as Parkinson's Disease and Alzheimer's Disease.

Cognitive Science: All processes and intricacies of the human brain and mind remain the focus of the increasingly intense research stemming from both the Human Genome Project and the Human Brain Project. Besides the potential development of artificial intelligence, scientists are particularly interested in the collection, storage and use of information within the brain. Specifically, scientists want to irrefutably identify and describe the concept of "cognition," the vast array of human mental abilities and functions. All of them are related to "knowledge," the ability to understand, be familiar with and use information. Within the mind, data is used to keep focused and attentive to specific topics for a period of time, commonly called "paying attention." These characteristics, in turn, result in the various higher-level mental functions unique to humans. The most important of these include: memory and working memory; judgment and evaluation; comprehension; problem solving and decision making; reasoning and computation; the ability to create, decipher and interpret languages; and numerous other mental processes. Naturally, these multiple and intermingled abilities tie closely to numerous specific fields of scientific study or medical practices. Besides computer science, systemics and biology, other integral fields of study include education, psychiatry, linguistics, anthropology and philosophy. To define or measure the levels of these characteristics, people usually use the concepts of "mind" and "intelligence."

Artificial Neural Network: Inspired by the ongoing analysis and discoveries of the human body's central nervous system, a massive network of machines--primarily computers-- would simulate the interconnected systems of biological neurons. These systems would be based on mathematical models, requiring an extensive and complex process, enabling researchers to conduct experiments. These tests would strive to analyze various biological theories involving the body's critical formation of proteins, and also studying the interactions and functions of neural systems within people. Scientists say that artificial neural networks have already been used to perform tasks such as speech recognition, and also generating the ability of "sight" in which machines understand, analyze and process images.

Artificial Intelligence: This highly specialized effort strives to achieve precisely what the term indicates, developing and creating machines that exhibit and actually use an artificial form of intelligence. Such a lofty goal hails as a monumental task, because animals--particularly humans--have a diverse, complex and highly specialized form of intelligence. Using the groundbreaking discoveries of DNA and the Human Genome Project as a basis, the machines would need the ability to communicate via natural languages--while also able to learn, plan, and to retain knowledge. All these should be done while also gradually or automatically developing a sense of reasoning or logic. Although such attributes remain a lofty hope for researchers, their current long-term goals focus primarily on what scientists call "general intelligence," the basic abilities of solving problems and perhaps reasoning. Scientists keep trying to coordinate the use of tremendous amounts of data from a variety of research disciplines. Ultimately, significant advancements in computer science seem to keep clicking these overall efforts into overdrive, marking the apparent start of technological developments that mankind has fantasized about for thousands of years. Besides general intelligence, other long-term goals include the development of "social intelligence"--the ability to interact effectively with others, and also the unique and often helpful ability that people have to use creativity in their everyday thought processes. Machines with such abilities have been the focus of many fictional works of literature and film, ranging from the "Terminator" movies featuring former California governor Arnold Schwarzenegger, to "Star Wars" and "Battlestar Galactica." Like this or not, a fear looms that the development of such machines could likely emerge as a "horror story come true," an irreversible scenario in which intelligent machines become strong, diverse and complex enough to destroy, control or rule humanity.

BRAIN Initiative: Striving to map the activity of every neuron in the human brain, in April 2013 the Obama administration announced the creation of the "Brain Research Through Advancing Innovative Technologies." Designed as a 10-year project costing $300 Million yearly, since its formation the BRAIN Initiative has been led by U.S. government laboratory scientists working in conjunction with the prestigious Allen Institute for Brain Science, the Howard Hughes Medical Institute, and the Office of Science and Technology Policy. Anyone who hates big government run amok, sometimes labeled the ultimate "Big Brother," might fear or detest such an effort. Yet the overall task is likely to also draw praise from people eager to achieve tremendous advances and better technologies made possible by Artificial Intelligence. According to various news reports, scientists started studying the brains of animals such as mice before advancing to humans. The initiative's success hinges on the successful development of nanoprobes used as electrophysiological multielectrode arrays, and nanoparticles used as voltage sensors to determine the electric potential difference between two points. This would measure the physiology of "action potentials," the brief electrical potential of a cell. Such a determination would be critical, enabling researchers to accurately and effectively measure what until now has been the highly complex, mysterious use of electrical impulses within the brain. When and if scientists are successful in reaching their goal of mapping every neuron within the human brain by mid-2023, at that point researchers would have the organ's equivalent of the human genome project map--a monumental event leading to additional technology.

Brain-Related Overview

The future of humanity looks either good or bleak in regard to genomics brain-studies stemming from the Human Genome Project.

On one side of the issue, proponents hope new advancements and technology will benefit humanity, improving the health of most people while also leading to the use of efficient machines.

Conversely, a well-grounded fear might arise when and if--as previously indicated--machines with Artificial Intelligence begin to "take over and rule the world."

By delving deep into the secrets of biology and the schemes provided by Mother Nature, do scientists and governments supporting them run the risk of going too far?

Mindful of these legitimate concerns, what checks and balances--if any--will need to be set in place to prevent such a system from getting out of hand?

The question becomes paramount, whether mankind is going too far, overstepping its bounds.

Truly, time will tell while at least one outcome seems fairly certain: Humanity must adopt reasonable criteria and safety systems, guaranteed to block any evil effort to universally "use machines to take over the world and control people everywhere."

14
Virtual Physiological Human

Rather than target any one particular organ, and determined to concentrate on the "whole body" of people, scientists envision the development of what they call the "virtual physiological human."

If successful, such an effort would enable researchers to work collaboratively in investigating a "single complex system," in this case the entire human body.

As envisioned by its proponents, the "virtual physiological human" would eventually provide critical information integrated into computer models. Data would include the biochemical, physical and mechanical functions of an entire human body.

After putting this critical information into a universal system stored online, various institutions and organizations worldwide could share the data using a framework designed as:

Descriptive: As much as possible, medical institutions such as hospitals and laboratories would continually input and share data on the human body. The system would be designed to combine, share, organize and catalogue the information.

Integrative: Working collectively, doctors, researchers and scientists worldwide from multiple disciplines would continually analyze and develop hypotheses.

Predictive: Participants would input the information into computer models, using systematic networks that ultimately enable researchers to determine if their hypotheses or theories are "correct." Tests would be done in laboratories or clinical environments.

For all this to happen, scientists would have to place all their data into a digital format, covering all major specialties involved in the study and treatment of humans--primarily physiological, and anatomical information.

Striving to Help Doctors

The overriding, primary and ultimate goal of the overall "virtual physiological human" is to enable doctors to better serve their patients.

For this to happen, researchers say that they first need to create and maintain effective and efficient computer models.

From the view of scientists, success here can only happen if a "multi-scale" modeling system integrates the body's various physiological systems against different time and length scales. To ensure accuracy on an international level, participants also would have to input "patient-specific data" germaine to certain segments of the world population.

Just as important, a systematic approach is necessary to avoid any incorrect conclusion, a "false assumption" that the entire human organism is "merely the sum of its parts."

All along, in order to achieve eventual success, scientists say that the effort also needs to avoid merely studying and adding data on individualized biological systems--such as concentrating on the heart, or any other organ or bodily system.

Essentially, the developers or proponents of any "virtual physiological human" want what some doctors describe as a "whole body approach."

Efforts Accelerated

Scientists first launched this effort via the Physiome Project, also known as the IUPS Physiome Project, in 1997, just five years before researchers finished mapping the entire Human Genome. The term "IUPS" refers to the International Union of Physiological Sciences.

In general and fairly understandable terms, a "physiome" is the physiological dynamic or "state" of an organism. These features include information on the structure--data on its morphome, proteome, and genome characteristics.

A physiome essentially defines the relationships that the genome has with the entire organism, plus the way that the individual's genes function.

First introduced in 1993 by the IUPS's Commission on Bioengineering in Physiology, the effort to develop a virtual physiological human has accelerated on a worldwide scale. The overall task clicked into overdrive in 2006 when the European Commission began funding "STEP: Structuring the EuroPhysiome."

Until then, various physiome studies and research programs or initiatives worldwide were loosely connected. Largely as a result, the overall STEP project was able to build what some experts call as "consensus process." At least 300 participants or "stakeholders" include policy makers, clinicians, industry experts and researchers.

Major Steps Forward

Following the publication of a booklet on this project's findings, "Seeding the EuroPhysiome: A Roadmap to the Virtual Physiological Human," this overall effort blossomed into a much larger worldwide process.

Besides obtaining additional funding, the effort grew in scope thanks to various collaborative projects in China, Japan and the United States.

As a core target of the European Commission's "7th Framework Programme," the effort still has a long-term goal of developing patient-specific computer models designed to enable doctors to give better, more effective treatment.

Besides creating ways to prevent disease, participants want to develop a more holistic medical approach, personalize medical care, and reduce the number of experiments involving animals.

Collectively and individually, all these efforts seek to enhance patient safety, while increasing the efficiency of treatments. Just as impressive, combined with their more holistic or natural approach, researchers also want to develop ways to simultaneously and effectively treat multiple organs rather than a single bodily system.

Human Connectome Project

The Human Connectome Project strives to map out and categorize the entire function of the human brain, separate from and unrelated to the Blue Brain Project and the "virtual physiological human."

The five-year connectome project is a component of the U.S. National Institutes of Health, the federal agency loaded with administrators, doctors and officials connected to the mainstream medical industry--closely tied to Big Pharma.

By contrast, the Blue Brain Project and the "virtual physiological human" are each tied to the European Union, within a region of the world that embraces and champions natural or "holistic" remedies at a far greater rate than in the United States.

Could these simultaneous but separate U.S. and European efforts eventually diverge into vastly different realms, with the American project recommending only dangerous drugs--while scientists elsewhere strive for more natural remedies?

Also, along these lines an additional but equally important question emerges: Would U.S. residents be given access to any effective natural treatments that might eventually be identified and verified by the European efforts?

Arguably, when using the past performance of the mainstream U.S. medical industry as a guide, the future in this regard looks dismal. The potential threat of eventually being forced to take unnatural drugs leaves a bitter taste in the mouths of any American who prefers a holistic approach.

Federal Support Emerged

As a hard-driving federal agency ensconced within the primary overall Human Genome Project, the National Institutes of Health (NIH) announced in September 2010 that it would award two separate grants totaling $38.5 million.

A $30 million grant was awarded to a consortium led by the University of Minnesota and Washington University in Saint Louis.

The second grant of $8.5 million went to a consortium led by the University of California Los Angeles, Harvard University and Massachusetts General Hospital.

Although each of these educational institutions has a well-deserved positive reputation for professionalism, each is closely tied to doctors and professors who all have been taught since the beginnings of their careers that "drugs--rather than natural substances--are the one and only way to go."

Despite these somewhat disturbing factors, the Human Connectome Project has the noteworthy goal of amassing useful data from healthy brains.

Scientists hope this valuable initial data will eventually lead to improved methods for researching various catastrophic or life-altering brain-related diseases or conditions such as schizophrenia, Alzheimer's disease, autism, and dyslexia.

Focus on Connectomes

The project focuses on the form and function of neural connections within the brain called "connectome."

Hailed by some researchers as the "wiring diagram" within this essential organ, the connectome serves as the key operator and system of the brain's nervous system.

The two separate consortium working on the Human Connectome Project have different but related research tasks:

Minn-WU Consortium: Researchers are mapping the large brain systems using non-evasive imaging technologies, thanks to 1,200 volunteers from 300 families--pairs of twins along with their siblings. Scientists hope to map each person's functional and anatomical connections throughout each part of the brain. The researchers then would compare genetic data and connectomes of the identical twins to those same factors within fraternal twins. This way scientists hope to determine how the brain's circuitry is shaped by the environment and genes. Rather than focus on individual neurons, researchers insist that mapping large brain systems serves as the necessary key to making the comparisons. Besides Washington University and the University of Minnesota, other institutions contributing to this consortium are Advanced MRI Technologies, the University of California at Berkeley, and six other institutions including Oxford University. Officials promise that the results from this study eventually will be available to the public via a Web-based, open-source neuroinformatics platform.

Harvard-UCLA/MGH: These researchers are using diffusion Magnetic Resonance Imaging (MRI) to identify and map all of the brain's structural connections. In order to be successful, scientists say, the research must effectively track the motion of water within the brain. This way testers can view the critical substance called "white matter," actually long extensions of neurons, viewable thanks to an imaging method where these structures are easily seen in "sharp relief." To do this, the teams use the diffusion MRI, tracking the motion of water within the brain's fibrous long-distance connections. Such images have become possible thanks to a unique scanner described as up to eight times more powerful than conventional systems.

In a continual cooperative effort, the two consortia eventually will share their findings, primarily the data derived from their separate mapping efforts.

Additionally, both efforts will use a variety of tests to identify and better understand the relationship between behavior and brain connectivity.

15
Human Microbiome Project

Scientists in the Human Microbiome Project are striving to fully understand for the first time how microorganisms live, thrive and impact the surface and interior of the human body-- particularly the gastrointestinal tracts.

Every moment of each day, each living human hosts literally billions of microorganisms, including those that separately cause "good" reactions and "bad" symptoms within the digestive tract. Researchers also yearn to know much more about what effects these microscopic living creatures have on saliva, oral mucosa and the various layers of skin, including the surface of the intestinal tract.

The term "microbiome" refers to the aggregate of microorganisms living--and eventually dying--in all these areas of an individual living person. According to some scientists, the amount of individual microorganisms on and in one person outnumbers by a 10-to-1 ratio the total cells that are part of the individual's body.

Many doctors, particularly Homeopaths, believe that many specific types of microorganisms are helpful to the human body, such as aiding in digestion and helping with the absorption of vital nutrients. Scientists insist that they need to know far more specifics on what negative impacts some "bad" microorganisms might have on human health.

Adding to the urgency, a 2009 article in "Scientific American" introduced the emerging question of whether the apparent or possible decrease in certain microorganisms in nature has been detrimental to overall human health worldwide.

Collect Urgent Data

Remember, the Human Microbiome Project lacked any formal significant ties to the milestone Human Genome Project.

Yet eventually the data collected and analyzed in the genome effort could--and likely will--be used in studying and determining the impacts of microorganisms. With persistence, perhaps scientists will be able to find "cures."

For such efforts to generate optimal results, however, the majority of scientists will need to demonstrate a true "leap of faith"--never trying to rely solely on the development of harmful, artificial drugs.

Instead, just as is the case with the Human Genome Project, researchers involved in the microbiome effort should focus on the potential benefits of effective yet harmless holistic remedies provided by Mother Nature.

Launched as a $115 million, five-year project in 2008, the microbiome effort ended on schedule in 2013, when scientists released their findings in more than 190 peer-reviewed publications. Among the Human Microbiome Project's most notable goals was to explore the interaction between changes to the human microbiome and diseases.

Like all major similar projects, particularly the primary Human Genome Project, the microbiome effort worked to study how its research impacted social, legal and ethical issues. While such a lofty goal might seem nebulous considering the effort's apparent close ties to Big Pharma, this project still managed to identify 3,000 genomes of pure bacterial strains--five times more than the original goal of 600.

Significant Discoveries Occurred

Thanks largely to the microbiome project's focused efforts, the research made numerous fairly significant strides. These milestones cleared the way for more comprehensive future research and the eventual possibility of at least some new treatments. Among some of the most important developments:

Digestive systems: According to "Cellular Microbiology," researchers discovered factors differentiating microbiota within people with healthy digestive systems, compared to characteristics of microorganisms in individuals suffering from "diseased guts."

Moving pictures: A 2011 article in "Genome Biology" revealed that scientists had finally obtained time-lapse "moving pictures" of the human microbiome.

Beneficial bacteria: In another groundbreaking discovery, researchers determined that certain microorganisms actually stimulate the body's natural T helper 17 cells, playing a key role in autoimmune disease--which results from an abnormal immune response.

Dangerous soils: Researchers discovered and confirmed that within soil bacteria communities Verrucomicrobia has a previously unrecognized dominant role.

Arterial disease: Tests confirmed that a microorganism in the mouth called an "oral microbiota" has been linked to arterial disease, commonly called atherosclerosis.

Vagina problems: Researchers found factors determining the virulence potential of "Gardnerella vaginalis," which leads to a disease of the vagina, bacterial vaginosis.

Various diseases: Researchers determined that Neisseria, a pathogenic microorganism species, is involved in the transmission of certain potentially fatal diseases or conditions: sexually transmitted disease; septicemia, a potentially fatal whole body inflammation that sometimes results in catastrophic organ failure; and meningitis, an acute inflammation of membranes that surround the brain and spinal cord.

Essential Database Established

In conjunction with various coordinated articles published in "Nature," in mid-2012 the National Institutes of Health announced that a reference database had been established by the Human Microbiome Project.

From 18 female and 15 male volunteers, researchers collected 3,000 microorganism samples from bodily sites that included the mouth, stools, skin, nose, and vagina. Based on these samples, scientists estimated that 10,000 different microbial species occupy what medical experts call the "human ecosystem." When announcing that they had created the database, NIH officials also revealed that the project generated numerous "surprise" findings. Among them:

Survival: The extended lifespan of each person depends more on microorganisms for survival than the individual's own bodily genes.

Variety: Various microbial species provide specific functions that help the human body. For instance, numerous microbial organisms assist the body's fat digestion.

Evolution: The overall microorganism or microbial components within people gradually change over time. This, in turn, results in changes to a patient's symptoms or reactions to disease, thereby requiring doctors to change medications.

New Action Recommended

According to a 2013 article in "American Pharmaceutical Review," the research indicated a need to monitor microorganism environments where products are manufactured.

In addition, microbiologists within the pharmaceutical industry want to ensure that certain microorganisms deemed objectionable never enter non-sterile drug products.

Also, according to a research paper resulting from the Human Microbiome Project, scientists found a decrease in the vaginal microbiome of women preparing for birth.

Meantime, the project's testers discovered a "high viral DNA load" within the nasal passages of children suffering from unexplained fevers.

With little doubt the Human Microbiome Project generated significant findings.

But rather than merely "studying the issue," mainstream doctors, the medical industry and particularly Homeopaths must take decisive action to use this critically important new information to improve patient care and treatment outcomes.

16
The Human Proteome Project

Scientists now are poised to make tremendous findings about life-giving proteins.

These factors are especially critical because all life among humans and other animals hinges on proteins, which supply energy and also cover certain genes.

To accomplish this important task, officials have started the Human Proteome Project, launched by the Human Proteome Organization as a collaborative project.

Along with various industry partners, the organization is an international consortium comprised of academic institutions, government researchers and research associations that specialize in "proteomics"--the large-scale study of proteins.

Human Variome Project

Boosted by discoveries from the primary Human Genome Project, scientists launched a new effort specifically designed to determine what doctors call "genetic variation" among individuals within single or among multiple populations of a species.

The overall effort of the Human Variome Project has been hailed as significant, primarily because the combined research is designed to unlock secrets to the genetic material essential to what Charles Darwin first dubbed "natural selection."

The vast majority of researchers believe that specific traits within a species gradually evolve or change over time. For those who believe in "evolution," all living creatures ranging from whales to elephants gradually evolved from other species.

As previously stated, under this line of thinking humans are the product of evolution. Over millions of years people gradually got larger brains and began to stand erect.

Today, this process is more frequently called "selected

breeding," rather than "natural selection" when first proposed as a theory by Darwin in the late 1800s. Mutations gradually generate genetic variation, when the chemical structure of a gene permanently changes.

Significant Impact Occurred

Based at St. Vincent's Hospital and the University of Melbourne in Australia, in a combined effort doctors and researchers launched the Human Variome Project to determine how genetic variation has impacted health.

With varying degrees of success, a wide variety of separate and unrelated efforts individually worked to make these discoveries. Most projects post or update their findings on the Internet. But until the launch of the Human Variome Project these other efforts had varying degrees of completeness, without any formal affiliation with each other.

To strengthen the overall effort, the Australian officials established the Human Variome Project. Administrators designed this new system as a central project, while collecting data from the various efforts, encouraging continued research, and eventually devising methods to improve health care.

As a result, the Human Variome Project supported the creation of at least 571 gene-specific databases. The primary project clicked into overdrive in June 2006 when bio-informatics scientists met with researchers, diagnosticians, and geneticists to organize the initial team for the effort's founder, Professor Richard Cotton.

Although this initial phase received relatively little publicity at its onset, numerous huge international corporations and organizations collectively and individually showed their interest in this field of study by attending the conference.

Besides officials from at least 20 genetics organizations worldwide, participants included Google, the World Health Organization, the European Commission, the March of Dimes, the

U.S. Centers for Disease Control and Prevention, and many others.

Focused Effort Solidified

Upon collectively concluding that the overall project should be pursued for the betterment of mankind, officials proposed that the Human Variome Project should have a five-year, $60-million budget spending an average of $12 million yearly.

This project's administrators report that the focused collective effort is necessary to develop the essential databases, and informatics or "information science." Without these research and information-storage platforms, scientists would be unable to envision and create effective new treatments.

An ideal information system also maintains useful data ranging from details about health care systems to behavioral and social science.

Meantime, officials at a non-profit effort, the Centre for Arab Genomic Studies, have proposed working throughout the Arab World to identify and prevent genetic disorders that have been reported among populations in that region.

The Arab Centre has represented that region at the Human Variome Project, while also associated with the Sheikh Hamdan bin Rashid Al Maktoum Award for Medical Sciences. Founded in 1999, the award honors scientists worldwide who pursue medical research that serves the broader interests of humanity.

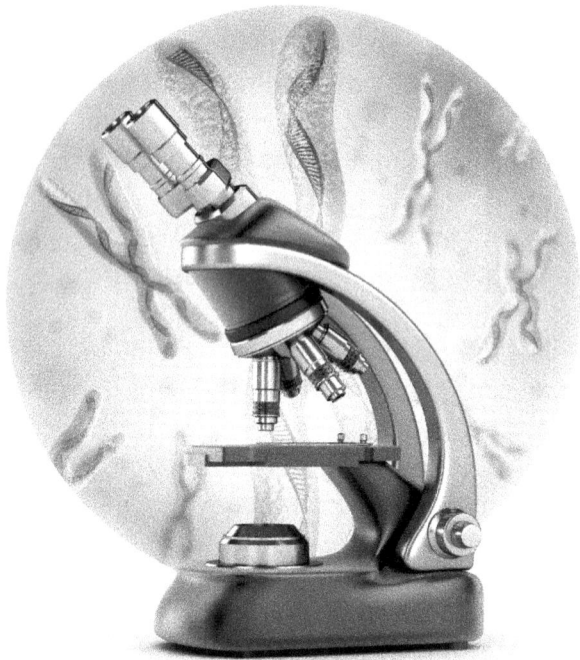

With a single blood sample and using a single affymetrix-based chip, scientists at the Genome Institute of Singapore have been able to detect 70,000 human pathogens including bacteria and viruses. The overall systems and technology developed by the company have become so effective and popular that numerous other firms have entered the competition in the DNA micorarray business.

17
Significant Systems Emerged

The massive and continually evolving worldwide efforts integral to genomics research motivated scientists to launch various individual--yet integrated--systems that are individually and collectively designed to improve the efficiency of research.

Almost as if a rapidly spreading helpful bacteria steadily encompassing the planet, many of these new systems were launched individually and independently of each other. Officials at these various efforts eventually found each other and entered strategic alliances. Among these efforts, organizations or formalized projects:

HUGO Gene Nomenclature Committee: Part of the Human Genome Organization (HUGO), this group strives to give a meaningful name deemed unique to literally every discovered human gene. To do this, the committee assigns an abbreviation, which scientists call "symbols," to each specific gene. As a result, researchers, scientists and medical facilities universally use the same identification system, which has various letters and numbers--each depending on the specific gene's individual characteristics and its placement within the overall human genome. Scientists insist that this naming or symboling system reduces potential confusion, with each symbol containing only Latin letters and Arabic numerals. The same symbols refrain from using the capitalized letter "G," the universal symbol for a "gene." In 2002, the committee first published its symbol guidelines, which have remained a medical industry standard. All along, the overall interrelated work of many differing genome research projects is so complex that when a program publishes a scientific paper, the committee contacts the author requesting the proposed nomenclature. The committee usually waits two weeks for a response, although time extensions are often granted. This process has become so extensive that the symboling system covers every type of species being studied. Meantime, in order to prevent possible confusion among scientists, the committee rarely approves changes to symbols initiated when a specific gene was first identified.

The Human Genome Organization: Often referred to as HUGO, this was launched in 1989, focused on helping scientists worldwide collaborate their efforts.

Affymetrix: A public company traded on the NASDAQ market under the symbol AFFX, the firm was founded in 1992 by Doctor Stephen Fodor. Based in Santa Clara, California, the company produces DNA "micorarray," which the general public commonly calls a "biochip" or a "DNA chip." Amazingly, these are solid surfaces that contain microscopic DNA spots. Biochips are extremely important to genomics research scientists. They use the devices in simultaneously measuring how large numbers of genes "express" themselves. This process called "synthesis" occurs when two or more genes meet together to form something new. These processes often involve proteins. Yet non-proteins also sometimes play an essential or integral role. Scientists use highly stringent conditions during research in order to accurately identify and describe test results. The incorporated affymetrix company, which typically avoids capitalizing the first letter of its name, went public in 1996. That initial public offering of stock occurred two years after the launch of the company's first product, the HIV Genotyping Gene Chip. The term "genotype" refers to the genetic makeup of a cell or organism. This process enables scientists to accurately and specifically identify the genomic characteristics of specific diseases ranging from HIV--the underlying cause of AIDS--to Cystic fibrosis and many other ailments. Since its launch, affymetrix has invented and created numerous microarray products, considered by scientists as necessary or highly preferable in conducting accurate, reliable research. By 2009 fiscal year revenues had reached $327 million. With offices and continental headquarters in the United Kingdom, Japan and China, the company produces some chips that can only be used once. A single chip can prove effective in simultaneously conducting thousands of experiments "in parallel." With a single blood sample and using a single affymetrix-based chip, scientists at the Genome Institute of Singapore have been able to detect 70,000 human pathogens including bacteria and viruses. The overall systems and technology developed by the company have become so effective and popular that numerous other firms have entered the competition in the DNA micorarray business. They include Agilent, GE Healthcare, Applied Biosystems, Beckman Coulter, and Illumina.

Research institutes: Dozens of respected, high-tech and cutting-edge human genomic research institutes have been launched worldwide since the entire human genome was finally mapped in 2003. Most independent, stand-alone institutions, these organizations have increasingly worked together to fine-tune and accelerate their overall progress. All continents except Antarctica are intricately involved to varying degrees. Besides hospitals, research facilities and university medical school laboratories, some are intricately linked to corporations. Just as impressive, many major governments or consortium of countries have given essential financial contributions to these efforts. The total contributions remain ongoing. These donations are incalculable in terms of human resources and actual dollars given--perhaps hundreds of billions of dollars and still growing. Within the United States, although linked closely to greedy Big Pharma, collectively and individually the various participating institutions have earned and deserve tremendous praise and the public's appreciation in these efforts. By recent count, every highly populated state's university system is involved from the East Coast to the West Coast. The institutions range from Stanford University in California to the University of Florida Genetics Institute in Gainesville, Florida.

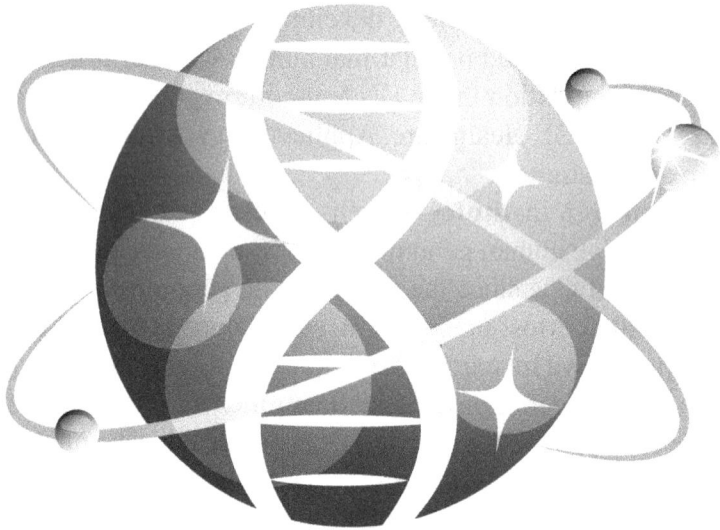

The 1,000 Genomes Project continues to progress as scientists search for ways to more specifically identify instances where a person is likely to eventually get a certain disease.

Numerous areas of biological science are expected to benefit, including bioinformatics, biochemistry, and pharmacology as scientists develop treatments and preventative remedies.

18
1,000 Genomes Project

Within a mere 2 1/2 years--from early 2008 to late 2010--
the all-encompassing 1,000 Genomes Project completed its pilot
phase in a quest to catalogue all human genetic variations.

In easily understandable terms, this entails detailing
and mapping the genetic differences among people in a
specific population, and other differences among various
separate populations. Variations in specific gene sets lead to
"polymorphism," a conditions that can generate completely
different characteristics within a single species although living
in a same population--sometimes even within the same overall
geographic area.

Many species experience polymorphism, ranging from
black, brown and white bears, to dark- and light-colored leopards.
For scientists studying humans, measuring and mapping the subtle
differences of such variations could lead to significant discoveries
necessary for the development of new treatments.

Such strides in medical technology can only occur after
studying these variations on a microscopic level--partly because
no two humans are precisely identical.

Target Alleles

In order for scientists to better understand these differences
they must unlock the secret to why and how the "alleles" or
genetic traits produce and exhibit physical characteristics at
different rates, levels and patterns.

For instance, several brothers with the same biological
parents might look fairly alike, but separately these males might
have varying shades of eye color.

Sadly, in the maturation of various organs and bodily
systems, such subtle and hard-to-decipher differences might lead

to a lifetime heart defect in one brother while all the others grow into healthy adults.

Potentially destructive variations also might emerge from specific gene characteristics, such as families where some females mature to have a greater propensity for developing breast cancer-- while related females never get the disease.

The 1,000 Genomes Project continues to progress as scientists search for ways to more specifically identify instances where a person is likely to eventually get a certain disease.

Numerous areas of biological science are expected to benefit, including bioinformatics, biochemistry, and pharmacology as scientists develop treatments and preventative remedies.

Pushing for Detail

Just beginning to understand how these subtle variations work, scientists are targeting two types of overall physical ailments. The first involves simple traits such as Cystic fibrosis and Huntington Disease.

Suspected of being associated with more complex traits, the other genetic variant likely create or lead to a biological environment or conditions that open destructive pathways for such ailments as heart disease, diabetes and cognition problems like dementias.

To emerge as successful, scientists must complete various specific tasks in laboratory settings. Among chores:

Large Scale Sequencing Network: Sequence at least 1,000 separate human genomes over a three-year period, before thoroughly analyzing results.

Tremendous Complexity: A mind-boggling estimated 10 billion bases would need to be sequenced or mapped daily during a two-year period.

Statistical Challenge: After amassing this basic level of necessary data, researchers would have a dataset comprised of a whopping 6 trillion DNA bases.

World-class Experts: To effectively process and analyze

the data, researchers will need the world's top experts in statistical genetics and bioinfomatics.

Separate Pilot Phases: Besides sequencing 1,000 genomes, scientists will need to map the genotypes of 180 people from three major genetic geographic groups, and also complete a deep-coverage sequencing study of two families--each comprised of biological parents with one of their adult children.

Life Needs Diversity

With increasing frequency in recent decades, scientists have begun to realize that all species of life need their own unique diversity in order to live and to thrive. As previously stated, Mother Nature commands that no two individuals of one species are 100-percent alike.

Plants and animals possess these subtle differences among each other, partly in order to help ensure that the species has a greater probability of surviving and thriving--particularly as environmental conditions gradually or rapidly change in subsequent generations.

Researchers want to use the 1,000 Genomes Project partly to better understand how the process of diversity works. Also, although most species gradually change over time, former or "extinct" predecessors of certain species have invariably disappeared.

Because of these factors, in a sense all life as a whole is gradually improving or adapting to help ensure that life continues in at least some form.

Throughout the entire living human population, genetic diversity occurs due to ongoing biological characteristics such as mutations and "copy-number variations" that result in differences in DNA that sometimes are abnormal.

Understanding Diversity

Ultimately via the 1,000 Genomes Project scientists are striving to get a far greater understanding of how natural selection works within the overall evolutionary process. To unlock these "secrets," researchers need more discoveries in each of the three classes of how evolution evolves on a DNA level:

Natural selection: How, why and when certain alleles within the genomic structure of each species have "greater fitness." When that occurs that allele--or biological trait--has an increased frequency within the overall population.

Negative selection: Working as the total opposite of "natural selection," the biological process of negative selection works to ensure that a species produces a decreased frequency of alleles deemed disadvantageous--when compared to other alleles.

Balancing selection: Associated with an increase in "genetic variation," some characteristics within a species can become over-dominant, thereby generating a biological condition where dominant characteristics or alleles block recessive characteristics. This leads to certain health problems such as the sickle cell anemia blood disorder.

Up to now, scientists have lacked a complete understanding of how these three genomic-level selection processes work, interact and progress through multiple generations. Yet the 1,000 Genomes Project might be on the verge of pinpointing the subtle variations in genes. Individually and collectively, these genetic differences give some individuals a variety of specific biological traits; they range from a greater resistance to certain diseases, to characteristics regulating responses to drugs.

19
Researchers Target Diseases

Working with massive amounts of information, scientific teams involved in the 1,000 Genomes Project want to better understand and cure ailments that result from complex biological conditions and from "Mendelian diseases," where biological features pass to subsequent generations.

Besides certain instances of Type 1 Diabetes, some of the most common culprits here include: Gaucher disease, a genetic conditions where too many fatty substances accumulate in certain organs and cells; Crohn's disease, an inflammatory bowel condition; and familial hypertrophic cardiomyopathy, where the heart's ability to contract decreases--usually leading to death.

The 1,000 Genomes Project strives to fill in what has been a significant gap in knowledge between two overall types of genetic variants related to disease. Scientists think that the most common type of variant stems from complex traits that result in conditions such as heart disease, diabetes and cognition problems.

The other least common type, labeled as "rare genetic variants," generates Cystic fibrosis and Huntington's Disease, a neurodegenerative genetic disorder that weakens cognitive abilities while changing behavior. People with Huntington's live an average of 20 years after their symptoms begin.

Sadly, many people with Huntington's disease have children long before the adults realize that they might have passed these destructive biological traits to their offspring. Advances in DNA technology should eventually enable people to determine if they're likely to develop Huntington's later in life.

Studying Specific Populations
To target specific diseases and genetic conditions, the overall 1,000 Genomes Project has been collecting genetic

samples from numerous specific segments of the worldwide population. Researchers launched these regional efforts because some negative biological traits that lead to disease are diverse within certain populations.

According to National Institutes of Health announcements issued in 2008, the regions where volunteers gave these DNA samples included: people in the Southwest United States of African ancestry; Los Angeles residents of Mexican ancestry; people of Chinese heritage living in metropolitan Denver; and Utah residents whose ancestors hailed from Northern and Western Europe.

Other sample-collection regions spanned such diverse locations as Nigeria, Tokyo, Beijing, Kenya, and the Tuscany area of Italy.

The results of studies on these samples, coupled with related work within the overall project, has generated valuable data used by scientists since 2012.

20
Personal Genomics Testing

The decreased costs and improved technologies of testing DNA have rapidly generated numerous services. Along with a reduction in overall costs, these factors have led to systems that enable individual consumers to get their personal genome tested.

Besides determining race and the probability of getting certain inherited diseases in later life, some specific testing services even enable individual consumers to get a definitive result on his or her projected life expectancy.

Costs of an individual "consumer test" have lowered significantly during the 2010s, to the point where some full tests are less than several hundred dollars.

Remember that as previously stated, starting at an average cost of $100,000 per individual in 2001, the total fees steadily and dramatically lowered to around $1,000--for instances where such tests are done on a full-blown level under the guidance of a physician or medical facility.

Fee decreases became possible thanks largely to improvements in systems used to measure, sequence and analyze the genomes within an individual.

Understanding Testing Methods

Consumers need to know the types and uses of such tests, even when done under the guidance and direction of a doctor. The two basic uses from a medical standpoint are:

Predictive medicine: Analyze and use the results to predict the probability that the individual will eventually contract certain diseases or ailments, before taking precautionary or preventative measures in an effort to block or minimize potential health issues.

Precision medicine: Target or identify existing conditions by using a unique DNA analysis, identifying the disease or health issue on a biological level before beginning targeted treatments.

As overall genomic testing and analysis techniques improve, heath care professionals would then identify everything from the specifics of cancer to the potential effectiveness of certain drugs and natural substances.

Potentially catastrophic diseases such as cancer ideally would be classified within a type or cause, before a battery of specifically pre-designed preventative treatments.

To maximize the probability of success, researchers and doctors would attempt to develop or identify the best type of drug--as indicated for each potentially destructive and unique genomic condition.

Rare Diseases Identified

According to the National Institutes of Health, about 200,000 people in the United States suffer from--or will acquire--some of the rarest diseases.

At least 2,500 illnesses stemming from genetic defects or DNA issues have been identified, all targeted through the "predictive genetics" analysis process.

So far, at least 11 companies or organizations specializing in individualized genomic testing have grown or started. Some of the most interesting include:

Life Technologies: Founded in 2008 and acquired in 2013 for $13.6 billion by Thermo Fisher Scientific, the Massachusetts-based company provides a variety of services and biotechnology products. Traded on the New York Stock Exchange under the trading symbol TMO, the company is considered one of the largest providers of precision laboratory testing equipment and genetic testing.

Pathway Genomics: This privately owned, San Diego-based company founded in 2008 by Jim Plante uses genetic testing to generate personalized reports specifying whether a person has an inherited genetic trait--indicating the development of certain complex diseases. These include hypertension,

Alzheimer's Disease, asthma, and many more. The company has registered its saliva collection with the U.S. Food and Drug Administration, listing the unit as an exempt medical device. The company's Website, Pathway.com, provides information on how its genomic tests detect cancer risks, cardiac health, carrier screening, weight management, and medication response.

23andMe: Via mail order, this Mountain View, California-based company provides direct-to-consumer, saliva-based test kits that use SNP Genotyping in measuring genetic variations. When sold to residents of Canada, depending on the type of test that the consumer orders, results can list the person's genetic risk of more than 240 diseases and potentially adverse health conditions, a process listed by "Time Magazine" as the Invention of the Year for 2008. Sadly, however, in 2013 the Food and Drug Administration allied to Big Pharma alleged that 23andMe had not obtained its legally required regulatory approval; the federal agency ordered the company to stop marketing its personal genome service. As a result, within the United States 23andMe still offers personal genome tests, but without health-related findings; U.S. users of the tests can only get results relating to their ancestral backgrounds. In Canada, however, the company is able to offer kits that generate results on ancestral data and medical information.

Physicians Required

As previously mentioned, anyone living in the United States who wishes to get a genomic test that lists their potential DNA-related diseases must do so only via a licensed physician, as mandated by the U.S. Food and Drug Administration.

This essentially means that within the USA the standard allopathic medical industry, in an association with a federal agency, essentially requires that patients must visit a doctor if they want to get such a test.

These restrictions became evident during the final three months of 2013, when--as previously mentioned--the FDA ordered the 23andMe service to end any and all marketing of that company's Personal Genome Service (PGS) and a Saliva Collection Kit.

An FDA document said that the agency is "concerned about the public health consequences of inaccurate results from the PGS device." Since then, within the United States, 23andMe has only sold ancestry-related results, plus broad genetic results.

Yet, the restriction would ultimately make little difference to consumers overall because other countries would provide open-source tools for analyzing such data, according to an November 2013 article in "Slate Magazine" by Rabiz Khan.

Criticisms Erupted

Unwilling to remain quiet on the issue, numerous health industry analysts and professionals quickly criticized the FDA's rule barring consumers from going anywhere other than physicians to get a long-term genomic diagnosis.

"The FDA bureaucrats think that they know better than you (on) how to handle your genetic information. This is outrageous," Ronald Bailey wrote in "Reason Magazine," a sentiment echoed by many others.

The behind-the-scenes debate featured numerous comments indicating that the FDA's stance is "ludicrous" because anyone discovering the likelihood of the onset of diseases later in life would likely seek the services of a licensed medical professional.

All along some observers took the opposite view, stating that firms such as 23andMe had allegedly failed to follow rules previously imposed by the agency.

In a November 2014 article for the Genetic Literacy Project, Arvind Suresh noted that what consumers learn from such tests "can sometimes be dangerous, because you may be getting vague, unhelpful or sometimes even false information from companies. What's worse is that in the short-term, this may cause the bubble of personal genomics to burst, setting back the rollout of truly revolutionary technologies."

Side-Stepping the Issue

Since the 23andMe issue erupted numerous companies have side-stepped the issue by offering genomics-related disease prognosis or analysis tests--yet only when ordered via a licensed physician.

"Some in the U.S. work around the FDA by offering these tests through physicians, an approach that does not require FDA approval, and is based on the assumption that practitioners can reliably evaluate the efficacy and interpret the results of these tests," Suresh's article said.

As such controversies and multiple options emerge, consumers should remain fully cognizant of the fact that the overall technologies involved undergo continual updating.

Indeed, although far more is know about genomics than a mere two decades ago, so much is still being learned on an almost daily basis that the process likely will continue for many more years before scientists begin reaching a consensus.

At present many researchers are more concerned with fitting together the entire puzzle--developing a far greater understanding of DNA processes--than starting out their testing procedures by immediately looking for a "cure."

As with any product or service, consumers considering such tests should do so with a "buyer beware" attitude. People need to remain mindful of the fact that if any adverse long-term prognosis results from such a test, a chance remains that little or nothing can be done--or, perhaps even worse, that results might emerge as "flat-out wrong."

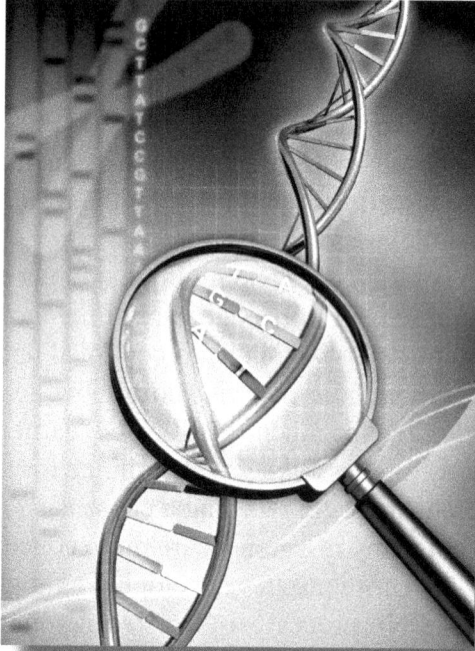

Thanks to numerous genetics study programs, medical professionals have been able to identify specific genes responsible for how the body metabolizes and responds to drugs. Building on research previously conducted as far back as the mid-1900s, scientists have identified various enzymes prevalent in the body that actively metabolize pharmaceutical products.

21
Creating New Drugs

Continually motivated to always generate new processes while making additional discoveries, scientists have developed systems for identifying and developing new drugs or treatments-- all possible thanks to genomic research.

The generic term for this drug- and treatment-creation process is called "pharmacogenomics," a combination of the words pharmacology and genomics.

Herein rests a potentially controversial and formidable issue, at least from the view point of anyone embracing the benefits of natural treatments as opposed to the development and use of unnatural and potentially dangerous drugs.

The overall process can emerge as highly complex when identifying and creating such products or substances. Researchers need to include numerous interrelated factors, including how the body absorbs, distributes, metabolizes and eliminates each substance.

With equal emphasis, within the body scientists need to identify the biological "receptor," a location that accepts and processes the substance.

Consumers and even some researchers need to realize there are differences between the terms "pharmacogenomics" and "pharmacogenetics"--although some medical professionals sometimes use these words interchangeably. The specific meanings are:

Pharmacogenomics: Viewed from a gene-wide perspective or approach, this deals with the responses of multiple genes. It incorporates genomics and "epigenetics," the biological study of physiological and cellular traits that are not caused by changes in the DNA sequence. Scientists target the stable but long-term potential of a cell to alter or interact with a substance.

Pharmacogenetics: This concentrates on a cell's interactions with a single drug.

Use Critical Data

The overall drug-creation process becomes extremely complex due to the massive quantities of genomic- or DNA-related information involved.

Doctors ultimately want to administer substances deemed highly effective, yet with minimal adverse side effects. For that to happen, research teams are busy identifying the specific genotype of individual patients--labeling or mapping the makeup of specific cells and organs.

Yet due to the specific nature of each person's unique DNA makeup, a vital concern erupts. Pharmacogenomics is unable to identify or create "one-size-fits-all" drugs for each ailment or disease caused by unique genetic factors.

On the positive side, according to a 2009 article in "Clinical Biochemistry Review," the development of genetic-generated drugs for each patient's specific needs would eliminate any "trial and error" when prescribing medications.

Ideally, this would emerge as the premiere and much-preferred form of "personalized medicine." Physicians would take into account the patient's unique genetic makeup when identifying a specific drug or combinations of drugs.

Vital Genes Identified

Thanks to numerous genetics study programs, medical professionals have been able to identify specific genes responsible for how the body metabolizes and responds to drugs.

Building on research previously conducted as far back as the mid-1900s, scientists have identified various enzymes prevalent in the body that actively metabolize pharmaceutical products.

The most prevalent include Cytochrome P450, a term first coined in 1962 and sometimes called "CYPs." These comprise a superfamily of "heme" containing a chemical compound--a tightly or covalently bound coenzyme. CYP enzymes are so prevalent that all known forms of life contain them, ranging from plants to animals and many additional domains including bacteria and even viruses.

CYPs are responsible for the metabolism of at least 80 percent to 90 percent of drugs already prescribed.

Besides Cytochrome P450, scientists have identified many other types of CYPs, including five that researchers test far more frequently than the others. Thanks to this research, medical professionals already know which overall types of drugs metabolize within specific forms of CYPs.

Noteworthy Goals Emerged

Pharmacogenomics researchers have developed numerous noteworthy goals. These can only be achieved by using what scientists already know about the efficacy or useful metabolism of certain drugs, while incorporating those essential details with vital information gleaned from new genomics discoveries. Among efforts described in a 2008 Humana Press publication:

Effectiveness: Prove that certain medications work

Best doses: Identify optimal dosing after determining a patient's unique genetic disposition to a specific drug

Improve: Maximize the discovery and development of effective new drugs

Safety improvements: Develop safer drugs with minimal adverse side effects

These overall efforts cover a vast array of medical areas ranging from psychiatry to oncology, pain management, cardiology and many other specialties.

Pharmacogenomics technology has become so advanced that researchers believe such science might eventually determine the specific cause of death from suspected fatal drug-related overdoses after autopsies fail to reach conclusions.

Also, as previously mentioned, genomics research has determined which patients are more likely to respond to certain types of cancer drugs--although the vast majority of mainstream oncologists in the United States ignore this critical and essential tool.

Too Many Drugs

Ideally, those of us concerned with the over-prescription of drugs in the United States want to remain optimistic that genomics will lessen the need for pharmaceuticals.

At the very least Pharmacogenomics should strive to eliminate or minimize "polypharmacy," the simultaneous prescribing of multiple drugs to individual patients. On a population-wide demographic scale, average seniors older than 65 seem to take far more prescription medications than any other age group.

Common sense dictates that although the bodies of some patients seem to react fine when simultaneously using numerous drugs, doctors should still do their utmost to minimize such instances.

The U.S. Food and Drug Administration seems highly invested in pharmacogenomics, according to a 2006 report by the European Commission's Joint Research Center's Institute for Prospective Technology studies. Just three years after scientists finished mapping the entire human genome, at least 160 drugs distributed in the U.S. markets already had pharmacogenomics biomarkers on their labels--a total that has surely grown since then.

Unique Challenges Emerged

The research, identification and development of drugs from genomic research has generated a set of unique challenges never previously faced by scientists and the medical industry. Based on various research reports and a survey by the Center for Genetics Education, various issues of concern to physicians and U.S. consumers include:

Access: Many doctors mention their apparent inability to access research and testing results

Knowledge: A failure to understand how physicians can

use the genomic test results in their clinical practices and when choosing treatments

Society: Concern about how ethical, legal and social issues will impact the doctors' decision-making process, an overall issue mentioned earlier

Providers: A lack of information regarding where and how to get genomic tests performed on individual patients

Collectively and individually, these issues should be a major concern to all practicing physicians. Most current doctors attended medical school well before the advent of today's steadily advancing genomic-based medical technologies.

Other Concerns Emerged

Locked into their current employment situations and restricted clinical environments, many medical professionals within Homeopathy and mainstream medicine find themselves faced with two additional primary concerns involving pharmacogenomics:

Insufficient scientific data: Besides the previously mentioned fact that most doctors lack details about pharmacogenomics tests, the majority of physicians have no access to critical all-encompassing scientific data on the metabolic pathways of such drugs.

Financial concerns: At least one report also indicates that publications issued by the pharmacogenomics industry are scarce. This signifies an apparent failure by various genomic researchers to distribute information on the potential cost effectiveness of such testing--plus data on total expenses.

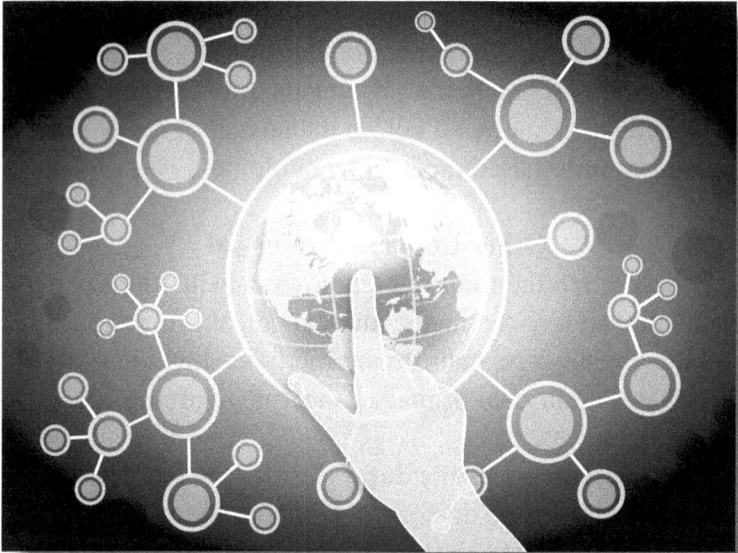

By the time officials launched the $3 billion
Human Genome Project in 1990, an international
consortium of geneticists had joined in the collective
effort. Scientists joined from such diverse places as
Japan, Australia, France and the United Kingdom.

22
Historical Considerations

In the wake of considerable DNA research and discoveries through the mid-20th Century, in 1987 American doctor Alvin Trivelpiece became the first physician to propose launching the Human Genome Project.

Trivelpiece's concept became possible thanks to the individual and collective efforts of numerous physicians and researchers from the 1950s through the mid-1980s.

One of the most significant developments leading to this landmark proposal occurred in 1985, when physicians and researchers met at a scientific workshop to discuss the human genome. Yet amazingly at the time, according to at least some published reports, the National Institutes of Health lacked interest in such an effort.

By 1986 officials from the U.S. Department of Energy's Office of Health and Environmental Research (OHER) organized an additional workshop, undaunted and determined to move forward with research and to share data from previous studies.

Meantime, scientific interest in DNA and genomics had intensified to the point that additional doctors and officials pressed forward with more professional gatherings organized to bolster and improve research.

Key Policy Maker
At the time Trivelpiece served as Assistant Secretary of Energy in the administration of President Ronald Reagan. A pivotal event occurred when OHER Director Charles DeLisi sent a memo outlining the project to Trivelpiece.

This document launched a series of bureaucratic and political events that culminated in a landmark event in scientific history in 1988, upon the initial congressional approval of a $16 million line item budget for the Human Genome Project.

Besides the strong proposal by Trivelpiece, the effort gained political traction when DeLisi befriended a key legislator, U.S. Sen. Pietro Vichi "Pete" Domenici, a New Mexico Republican who served in the Senate from 1973 to 2009.

When viewed on a grand scale, these various scientific and political events were timed perfectly, partly thanks to the fact that by 1985 researchers already had compiled a fairly extensive list of technologies--each listed as candidates for much-needed research.

Unusually efficient considering the fact that each is a giant federal bureaucracy, in 1990 the U.S. Department of Energy (DOE) and the National Institutes of Health (NIH) mutually agreed on a memo of understanding on how to coordinate plans for the Project.

On the strength of these efforts, coupled with the fact that funding had been secured, officials started the formalized Human Genome Project effort that year.

Efforts Became Increasingly Focused

Within several months the NIH had launched its Genome Program, while the DOE started the Office of Biological and Environmental Research.

By the time officials launched the $3 billion Human Genome Project in 1990, an international consortium of geneticists had joined in the collective effort. Scientists joined from such diverse places as Japan, Australia, France and the United Kingdom.

Officials streamlined the effort further in 1993 when Francis Collins became Project Head at the NIH's National Human Genome Research Institute.

Soon ahead of schedule thanks to intense and effective international cooperation and technological advancements, in the year 2000 scientists completed what they considered a "rough" draft of the entire human genome.

Scientists at the University of California, Santa Cruz's Genome Bioinformatics Group submitted this critical data, clearing the way for the 2003 completion of the entire human genome map. This milestone occurred two years earlier than what officials had originally anticipated in 1990 when first launching and approving the project.

Proposed Benefits Identified

From the start, scientists identified and started targeting a vast array of scientific fields likely to benefit from this groundbreaking research.

First and foremost, at least from the perspective of the general public first learning basics overall details, the overall effort seeks to identify and "cure" disease.

Yet the overall research and the technological advancements that occurred as a result are much more far-reaching than many people realize. The most critical areas include:

Energy: The development of biofuels and other potential energy sources.

Viruses: Genotyping viruses, partly in order to develop effective treatments.

Cancer: As previously mentioned, identify mutations and oncogenes, leading to cancer "cures" or drugs.

Forensics: Advancements in applied sciences, leading to improvements in genomic research and also technology vital to criminal investigations.

Medications: Genomic discoveries leading to the creation or development of effective drugs or treatments.

Multiplicity: The eventual development of technology boosted numerous business sectors and scientific areas. These range from bioprocessing, risk assessment and agriculture, to livestock breeding, evolution, anthropology, and duplicated bioarcheology.

Multiple Simultaneous Efforts

In order to continually and efficiently push forward with all these efforts on a collective and individual basis, in the meantime scientists working in conjunction with major universities and research institutions have needed to create:

Databases: Available to anyone accessing the Internet, these sites store voluminous amounts of critical information vital to essential advancements in genomics.

Governments: The U.S. government launched the National Center for Biotechnology Information, to implement, disseminate and maintain the databases, in cooperation with sister organizations in Japan and Europe,

Unique Browser: While continually playing an important role in genomics research and data dissemination, the University of California, Santa Cruz, created the UCSC Genomic Browser. This interactive Website hosted by the university gives access to genomic research data from a variety of species including vertebrate and invertebrate.

National effort: The National Institutes of Health's National Center for Biotechnology Information houses a series of databases involving biomedicine and biotechnology, founded in 1988 and based in Bethesda, Maryland. The agency's significant databases include PubMed, a bibliographic database storing biomedical literature, and GenBank, which specializes in DNA sequences.

Europe: On an equally important basis, the European scientific community launched "Ensembl," a joint scientific project between the Wellcome Trust Sanger Institute and the European Bioinformatics Institute. Launched in 1999, Ensembl provides a centralized source for researchers studying the human genome, model organisms and other vertebrates.

23
Rapid-Fire Advancements Occur Daily

Significant or amazing developments in the genomics industry and research clicked into overdrive on a daily basis by late 2014, seemingly "faster than a speeding bullet" just like the fictional super-hero Superman.

By then many major and compelling studies and new findings were being steadily announced, accelerating to the point where most genomic discoveries failed to get any significant mention in the mainstream news media.

A stark realization became crystal clear for almost anyone eager or willing to follow these developments. Scientists had entered a brave new realm, proclaiming that within several years that they actually would be able to recreate dinosaurs.

Amazingly, however, the average person seemed oblivious to such sensational claims, which scientists swore that they could back up with verifiable data.

If even a fraction of these predictions once thought to be outlandish emerge as "true," then average consumers everywhere are soon destined to experience significant changes in their lives-- meeting or surpassing how the Internet has changed society.

Pay Close Attention to Discoveries

Everyone needs to pay far closer attention to the daily advancements in genomics, thereby enabling themselves and their families to prepare emotionally and financially for the significant social and medical changes that are on the verge of becoming "reality."

The following advancements, discoveries or predictions deserve to remain high on the news media radar:

Everyone listed: According to numerous news agencies, the entire genomics map of each living person on earth could be

143

stored in an online cloud by Google--by far the world's largest and most profitable online Web-based company. Without seeking publicity or announcing these efforts, by late 2014 the company had already been quietly moving forward with this project called "Google Genomics." Some analysts apparently considered such an effort to store the DNA map of each of the living 7 billion people on earth as impossible, considering the massive amounts of data storage required. Such skepticism might seem understandable, considering the fact that each person's body has billions of unique DNA signatures. Despite such obstacles, scientists already have proven that what the general public once thought as "impossible" is actually "reality." Although little has been revealed about Google Genomics, some researchers view that company's efforts as the key to unlocking and launching a pivotal international genomic database. When at an efficient and economically viable level, such a database system--in turn--could eventually lead to groundbreaking medical advancements of earth-shattering impact.

Human mating decisions: Some scientists believe that at least half of all people carry certain DNA characteristics that could prove fatal to their offspring--if the children are sired by a mother and father, each with similar negative genomic characteristics. According to a "Forbes" article written by David Shaywitz, Chief Medical Officer at a cloud-based genomic data management platform, DNAnexus, many people seem understandably worried that having a personal genomic test might indicate the likelihood or potential onset of a serious--perhaps fatal--ailment later in life. "Yet, there's another approach to genetics that is recently gaining traction, a methodology that seems to look at the genome through a more hopeful and positive lens," Shaywitz wrote. "In this 'Happy Genetics,' the goal is to find people who are unexpectedly healthy, and then search for the genes potentially responsible."

Epilepsy discovery: The dreaded and much-misunderstood disease of epilepsy is just one of many afflictions that scientists have learned much more about thanks to genomics. The online "MedicalXpress" news service has reported that genomic researchers have discovered a new, previously unknown genetics cause for one of the most devastating forms of the disease, progressive myoclonus epilepsy. According to the report, a study by an international research consortium discovered a single mutation--an underlying potassium ion channel gene that "underlies a substantial portion of unsolved cases. It is estimated that the mutation is carried by hundreds of patients worldwide." The publication "Nature Genetics" released results of the study led by researchers at several universities in Finland and Australia. According to MedicalXpress, the findings could lead to "potential therapeutic interventions of the disease."

Human Testes: According to a report by the British Broadcasting Company, the Royal Institute of Technology in Sweden has identified the human testes as the "most distinct type of human tissue." The report said that the research team detailed specific proteins that "are active in which tissues of the human body. It showed the testes needed the most distinct site of proteins to function." This finding was reached by the Human Protein Atlas, which the BBC says has been described as a "'really important foundation' for scientific research that could help develop new drugs." In that process, the BBC said, scientists have mapped which types of proteins function in specific bodily areas, and "hope the findings could have important implications for medicine." The report said scientists identified 999 proteins that are significantly more active in the testes than anywhere else in the human body. By contrast, the report said, the "cerebral cortex of the brain had 318, the liver 172, and and smooth muscle zero."

Restructuring nature: Based on discoveries generated from the Human Genome Project, scientists have been attempting to create pigs that possess and function with lungs identical to those organs in humans, according to a story published by the "San Jose Mercury News." The report said that scientists want to generate this unique form of pig, in order to use the animal's humanlike lungs for people needing the organs in transplants. The story quoted Craig Venter, a genome pioneer at the "SynBioBeta" company as saying "we are re-engineering the pig, changing its genetic code. If we succeed with rewriting the pig genome, we will have replacement organs for those who need them." Venter said that scientists already were using computers needed to create the code, necessary for building the hybrid. For many years, doctors have been using parts of pig hearts for use in operations to repair the human aorta. Hopefully, improvements generated by genomics research can maximize the efficiency and success of such procedures. Of particularly concern is eliminating the need for viable heart transplants, the current process of using the organs of people killed in accidents or homicides.

Military defense applications: According to reports disseminated by various news media outlets, the U.S. government allotted $1 million from a defense appropriations bill to Schott North America. The company agreed to use the funds to develop what the "GenomeWeb" service called a "macroarray-based platform for detecting biological agents." The system will be designed to detect up to 2,000 potentially harmful biological pathogens.

Cancer Drugs: According to the Boston-based WBUR news station, "scientists say they are on the verge of developing a greater number of treatments for cancer that are more efficient and less toxic, by specifically targeting tumors using genetic analysis." The story quoted Doctor Edward Benz, president of Dana-Farber Cancer Institute, as saying that "we've already developed dozens of new drugs that are not like the carpet bombing of chemotherapy. They're much more like smart bombs." Benz told WBUR that among humans, cancer is an incredibly common disease, and "that's why people are dying from it." Benz lists the aging process, particularly in mature individuals, as the biggest risk factor for cancer--resulting in a greater overall number of instances as the population ages. Yet thanks to genomic advances since 1999, scientists are now beginning to target the root causes of cancers that stem from changes in the genome. When that happens, Benz said, genomic changes cause some genes to "go bad," accelerating the growth of cancerous cells. He predicts that new cancer-fighting drugs developed as a result of the genetics research will make the use of chemotherapy less common.

More Cancer Targeting: Leading to additional breakthroughs in the fight against cancer, medical genetics researchers remain busy discovering why and how the cell replication process typically becomes disrupted in patients suffering the disease. According to the MedicalXpress news service, a Florida State University research team "is pushing the limits on what the world knows about how human genetic material is replicated and what that means for people with diseases where the replication process is disrupted, such as cancer." Quoting the journal "Nature," the MedicalXpress report said that a paper by the research team indicates that future advancements from the tests can lead to breakthroughs. As part of a multi-university effort, the report said, researchers studying mice genomics in comparison to human DNA are closely examining the replication process "so they could identify the units by which the genetic material replicated. They knew it happened at regular intervals, but they needed to know what the boundaries were." David Gilbert, a Department of Biological Sciences professor at the Florida institution, said that that scientists successfully identified the units of replication, a "fundamental first step in identifying a new phenomenon in nature."

Renal Cancer: Scientists have finally developed a better understanding of the genetic mysteries of renal cell carcinoma, after previously developing discoveries unlocking the attributes of numerous other malignancies. According to "Medpage Today," the findings have enabled scientists to discount a previous viewpoint that incorrectly assumed that all tumors are alike. The report quoted a researcher as indicating that as recently as the 1980s doctors incorrectly believed that essentially all cancers were "a single disease, resulting in a process where all cancer patients were surgically treated the same."

Superdrugs: Thanks to significant advancements in genomics research, scientists were on the verge of developing to "superdrug" to eradicate dangerously high cholesterol levels among people worldwide, according to the Massachusetts Institute of Technology (MIT). The burst in development for the new pharmaceutical came after researchers discovered that many people worldwide are missing a basic gene called PCSK9, individuals who had "almost no bad cholesterol in their blood," said the "Technology Review," an MIT publication. Striving to benefit from this unique characteristic, researchers developed a drug capable of disabling the gene's activity. "People taking the medications have seen their cholesterol levels plummet dramatically, sometimes by 75 percent," the review said, adding that the new pharmaceutical developed by Regeneron Pharmaceuticals was nearing FDA approval. The report also says that "by in large, it's not good to be missing a gene. Yet missing a gene can sometimes provide powerful protection against disease."

Homosexuality: Thanks to advancements in genomics research, scientists have been able to identify a "potential genetic cause for homosexuality," according to a "Latin Post" news report. "Though the study is not considered precisely conclusive, it brings scientists closer to finding a genetic connection to homosexuality in human males." Described as the largest study of its kind to date, the project's findings were based on information gathered from 409 pairs of "homosexual brothers." According to the "Post" story, "Discover Magazine" had described the study as involved in both "x chromosome and chromosome 8, which has been discovered to (be) related to male sexual orientation." The item said that researchers collected saliva and blood samples from pairs of brothers, which included twins. While studying various specific genomic markers from among the test samples, researchers noted that the brothers all were gay, although individuals within these pairs had differing characteristics including height, hair color and intelligence levels. The report said that amid research two genetic markers appeared most frequently-

148

-the Xq28 region of the X chromosome, and the 8q12 region of the 8 chromosome. This has "led scientists to believe it is connected to male homosexuality." Despite these reports, as reported by the Associated Press there have been some skeptics, including Neil Risch, a University of California, San Francisco, genetics expert who called the data "statistically too weak to demonstrate a genetic link."

Platinum Genome: Although researchers in 2003 declared the completion of mapping for the entire Human Genome Project, scientists have admitted since then that literally hundreds of sequences in the DNA map had not actually been finished. This intentional oversight remained a problem; some genetic markers overlooked by these intentional oversights have been linked to disease. At the time the mapping was actually only 99-percent complete due to limitations in methodology. Determined to close the gap while "filling in the blanks," thanks to significant advancements in research technology since 2003, several genomic mapping projects have approached near-completion, a status called the "Platinum Genome." "It's like mapping Europe and somebody says, 'Oh, there's Norway. I really don't want to have anything to do with fjords. Now, somebody is in there mapping the fjords," a microbiologist at the European Bioinformatics Institute, Ewan Birney, told the publication "Nature." As a result of these persistent Platinum Genome efforts, "Nature" says, scientists are getting a greater understanding of autism and neo-degenerative diseases like amyotrophic lateral sclerosis (ALS).

Human Interactome: Much more still needs to be know about the connections of genotypes and phenotypes, regardless of the significant medical industry and research advancements made possible by the Human Genome Project. To fill in this knowledge gap, according to the publication "Cell," the Human Interactome Map is being developed by the Center for Cancer Systems Biology, at the Dana-Farber Cancer Institute. Fritz Roth of the University of Toronto, co-author of the study, told that publication that "this is a long road, and we've never had a human interactome project to go with the Human Genome Project. But I think that people are starting to appreciate that the genome is the beginning of the story--it's a parts list in an alien language that we're starting to figure out." To push forward with this effort, Roth said, researchers have been using what they call a "yeast two-hybrid system"--measuring "two different configurations for their ability to activate a reporter gene in yeast." The report said that as a result scientists were able to use a "systematic strategy that picked up a large swath of interactions that were missed by individual studies." Since those landmark findings began in 2010 researchers have continued developing subsequent Human Interactome maps.

Brain Tapeworms: In 2014 doctors surgically removed a mysterious and extremely rare centimeter-long parasitic tapeworm from the brain of a Chinese man who had been experiencing neurological disorders during the previous four years. Curious researchers completed a genomic sequence of the creature, marking the first time such a species had undergone such a procedure. According to the "PopSci" online publication, researchers hope the worm's genetic information will "help clinicians better diagnose and treat this parasite infection and others like it in the future." Scientists revealed that the creature, with the scientific name "Spirometra erinaceieuropaei," eats by absorbing fats through its skin; lucky for the worm, fats are abundant in the human brain.

24
Who Owns the Human Genome?

Although most Americans remain unaware of such a major development, the United States Supreme Court made a landmark 2013 decision--proclaiming that companies or people are unable to own all or part of the human genome.

This unanimous landmark ruling involved a civil court case between two U.S. companies, each claiming the ownership of patents on two genes that scientists believe are frequent causes of breast and ovarian cancer. The jurists used a common-sense approach, concluding that such patents are unlawful because genes are a product of nature.

The ruling came 13 years after former President Bill Clinton issued an executive mandate in 2000, ruling that the genome sequence could not be patented.

Clinton's decision came two years after a former National Institutes of Health scientist, Craig Venter, and his Celera Genomics firm launched a project similar to the Human Genome Project. Celera's effort was privately funded for $300 million. Venter's effort attempted to beat the $3 billion U.S. government-funded Human Genome Project in finishing a full map of the human genomic sequence.

According to an August 2013 article issued by the Center for Biomolecular Science and Engineering, Celera had filed patent applications that would have given the company ownership of at least 6,500 partial or whole genes.

Results of This Justifiable Ruling
The Supreme Court ruling resulted in numerous positive outcomes for consumers, patients and the scientific community:

Avoid Confusion: Streams of companies legally battling over ownership to specific genes could have generated substantial confusion. Such situations that likely would have slowed or even blocked vital ongoing research efforts.

Consumer Protections: People worldwide never had situations where they would need to say things such as: "XYZ Acme Company owns all the genomes in my heart from the moment that I'm born until I die, while another firm owns my bones."

Cost Limitations: By essentially proclaiming that companies can actively compete for "cures" based on universally shared information regarding human genomes, the courts might have limited any company from imposing over-the-top fees.

Enthusiasm: Firms and educational institutions were now free to continue vital and extremely expensive DNA and genomic research tests without any fear that all such efforts might proverbially "go down the tubes."

Although all these various benefits are undeniably significant, consumers also need to keep in mind that companies still retain the right to patent and eventually profit from synthetic drugs developed as a result of genomic research.

25
Look to Century Wellness Clinic for Guidance

A giant, glaring and obvious question emerges from all this sensational and earth-changing information regarding genomic research: Why is my cancer treatment strategy and health clinic one of perhaps a mere handful of professional medical facilities in the United States to offer chemosensitivity tests?

With equal importance has emerged the disturbing and perhaps shocking revelation that virtually all mainstream oncologists refuse to offer such vital tests and even to admit that this tremendous technology exists.

To say that such tests are "extraordinary and capable of positively changing anti-cancer medicine forever" would be far from an understatement.

Well, with little doubt the key elements of this issue come down to political skulduggery throughout the medical system and governmental systems of our nation.

Does all this selfishness, greediness and heartlessness hinge on an unquenchable lust by mainstream doctors for money, power and a warped desire to control how people live--or even whether patients survive?

Frankly, I need to say without any reservations whatsoever that our nation's medical industry and government is embossed with varying degrees of corruption.

Take a Positive Stand

The non-stop migration by cancer patients to my clinic continues unabated, at least 1,300 Americans are dying from cancer every day.

Well before they perished, if all those patients were given chemosensitivity tests along with the type of natural remedy-regimens that I provide, at least 845 of those individuals would have survived for at least five years.

At that rate, by using the type of technologies that I provide, mainstream oncologists would collectively help save the lives of 308,425 Americans every year.

These totals become even more disturbing on a worldwide basis; millions of cancer patients could be saved around the globe every year if all doctors used the medical treatment strategies available at my clinic.

I Remain Ready to Serve

The doors to my medical facility remain open to all qualified patients.

As many consumers might very well imagine, the total number of patients served by Century Wellness Clinic has steadily increased in recent years.

At the time of this book's initial publication, "spaces" remained available for new patients. Yet for as long as demand continues to steadily increase for my services, getting a confirmed reservation in a timely manner is likely to become increasingly difficult.

So, I recommend that all potential patients, particularly those suffering from Stage IV cancer, inquire as soon as they would like about the possibility of making a reservation.

Keep in mind that cancer is far easier to "cure" when treated in early stages of the disease.

Accept Extraordinary Medical Advances

As my clinic's patient load continues to increase, I urge medical facilities worldwide, along with mainstream and Homeopathic doctors, to embrace and use cutting-edge genomic technology.

Although these rapidly progressing techniques and systems offer extraordinary potential, such processes will remain of little or no value unless doctors start to use them.

I respectfully proclaim to the entire medical profession that we all need to get our head out of the sand. Collectively and individually, we as physicians need to embrace and to use the best new genomic technology for the betterment of our patients.

This means that rather than insisting on and using a system that poisons and ultimately kills almost all worst-stage cancer patients, we need to--and we must--break the reckless bounds of mainstream protocol that requires mainstream oncologists to administer high-level, extremely toxic and poisonous chemo in all Stage IV cancer cases.

With equal urgency, while adhering to the Hippocratic oath specifying that all doctors must work for the best interests of patients, physicians everywhere must collectively strive to weaken the negative grip that Big Pharma has on all of society.

Working in conjunction with politicians, we can and should encourage the passage of laws restricting the amounts of campaign contributions that huge pharmaceutical companies dole out to political candidates.

All this should happen as governmental leaders work effectively to remove or ban Big Pharma allies from occupying the offices, leadership roles and staff-levels positions at governmental agencies that impact health--such as the Food and Drug Administration.

An additional effort should go toward ongoing government-funded genomic research, ensuring that those efforts strive to develop and to identify natural remedies--which always should be considered far more preferable than harmful, expensive and potentially addictive drugs.

Common sense, a love for humanity and compassion collectively and individually dictate that all types of physicians should work together to implement these vital measures.

We Remain Strong

Century Wellness Clinic's current and future patients can rest assured that the facility will continue offering chemosensitivity tests.

Steady and rock-solid, along with my staff I shall strive to maintain and even increase the clinic's already-superior cancer survival rates.

My clinic will continue its leadership role, especially for as long as mainstream doctors refuse to enable patients to benefit from phenomenal new genomic technology and effective, harmless natural remedies.

About the Author

James W. Forsythe, M.D., H.M.D., has long been considered one of the most respected physicians in the United States, particularly for his treatment of cancer and the legal use of human growth hormone. In the mid-1960s, Dr. Forsythe graduated with honors from University California at Berkeley and earned his Medical Degree from University of California, San Francisco, before spending two years residency in Pathology at Tripler Army Hospital, Honolulu. After a tour of duty in Vietnam, he returned to San Francisco and completed an internal medicine residency and an oncology fellowship. He is also a world-renowned speaker and author. He has co-authored, been mentioned in and/ or written chapters in bestsellers. To name a few: "An Alternative Medicine Definitive Guide to Cancer;" "Knockout, Interviews with Doctors who are Curing Cancer" Suzanne Somers' number one bestseller; "The Ultimate Guide To Natural Health, Quick Reference A-Z Directory of Natural Remedies for Diseases and Ailments;" "Anti-Aging Cures;" "The Healing Power of Sleep;" and "Compassionate Oncology ~ What Conventional Cancer Specialists Don't Want You To Know;" and "Obaminable Care," "Complete Pain," "Natural Pain Killers," and "Your Secret to the Fountain of Youth ~ What They Don't Want You to Know About HGH Human Growth Hormone," "Take Control of Your Cancer," "Understanding and Surviving Obamacare," "About Death from a Cancer Doctor's Perspective," "Dr. Forsythe's Whey Protein Anti-Aging Formula," and the "Emergency Radiation Medical Handbook."

Contact Information

Dr. James W. Forsythe, M.D., H.M.D.
Century Wellness Clinic
521 Hammill Lane, Reno, NV 89511-1004
775-827-0707
Website: DrForsythe.com
Email: RenoWellnessDr @ yahoo.com